SENSITIVE
GASTROINTESTINAL DISORDERS

FEDOTOZINE CONTRIBUTION
TO DRUG THERAPY

British Library Cataloguing in Publication Data
A catalogue record for this book is available from the British Library.
ISBN 2-7420-00

Éditions John Libbey Eurotext
127, avenue de la République, 92120 Montrouge, France
Tél : (1) 46.73.06.60

John Libbey and Company Ltd
13, Smiths Yard, Summerley Street,
London SW18 4HR, England
Tel : (1) 947.27.77

John Libbey CIC
Via L. Spallanzani, 11
00161, Rome, Italy
Tel : (06) 862.289

SENSITIVE GASTROINTESTINAL DISORDERS

FEDOTOZINE CONTRIBUTION TO DRUG THERAPY

**Proceedings of a symposium
held in Versailles,
December 5th 1994**

J.P. GALMICHE
B. FRAITAG

Contents

List of contributors

Abitbol J.L., Institut de Recherche Jouveinal, 3-9, rue de la Loge, 94265 Fresnes Cedex, France.

Asal K., Policlinique Médicale Universitaire, 19, rue César-Roux, 1005 Lausanne, Switzerland.

Azpiroz F., Digestive System Research Unit, Hospital General Vall d'Hebron, Autonomous University of Barcelona, 08035 Barcelona, Spain.

Bischof-Delaloye A., Policlinique Médicale Universitaire, 19, rue César-Roux, 1005 Lausanne, Switzerland.

Blum A.L., Centre Hospitalier Universitaire Vaudois, Lausanne CH011, Switzerland.

Borovicka J., Policlinique Médicale Universitaire, 19, rue César-Roux, 1005 Lausanne, Switzerland

Buéno L., Department of Pharmacology, INRA, Toulouse, France.

Coffin B., INSERM U 290, Hôpital Saint-Lazare, Paris, France.

Collins S.M., Intestinal Diseases Research Unit, McMaster University, Hamilton, Ontario, Canada.

Corazziari E., II Clinica Medica, Policlinico Umberto I, Università degli Studi La Sapienza, Cattedra di Gastroenterologia, 00161 Roma, Italia.

Dapoigny M., Service de Gastroentérologie, Hôtel-Dieu, 36003 Clermont-Ferrand Cedex, France.

Diop L., Institut de Recherche Jouveinal, 3-9, rue de la Loge, 94265 Fresnes Cedex, France.

Fraitag B., Institut de Recherche Jouveinal, 3-9, rue de la Loge, 94265 Fresnes Cedex, France.

Fraser R., Policlinique Médicale Universitaire, 19, rue César-Roux, 1005 Lausanne, Switzerland.

Fried M., Policlinique Médicale Universitaire, 19, rue César-Roux, 1005 Lausanne, Switzerland.

Galmiche J.P., Service d'Hépato-gastroentérologie, Hôpital Guillaume et René Laënnec, BP 1005, 44035 Nantes Cedex 01, France.

Gebhart G.F., Department of Pharmacology, College of Medicine, University of Iowa, Iowa City, IA 52242, USA.

Gué M., Institut de Recherche Jouveinal, 3-9, rue de la Loge, 94265 Fresnes Cedex, France.

Homerin M., Institut de Recherche Jouveinal, 3-9, rue de la Loge, 94265 Fresnes Cedex, France.

Jian R., Service de Gastroentérologie, Hôpital Saint-Louis, 1 avenue Claude-Vellefaux, 75010 Paris, France

Junien J.L., Institut de Recherche Jouveinal, 3-9, rue de la Loge, 94265 Fresnes Cedex, France.

X

Kreiss C., Policlinique Médicale Universitaire, 19, rue César-Roux, 1005 Lausanne, Switzerland.

Langlois A., Institut de Recherche Jouveinal, 3-9, rue de la Loge, 94265 Fresnes Cedex, France.

Lémann B., Service de Gastroentérologie, Hôpital Saint-Louis, 1, avenue Claude-Vellefaux, 75010 Paris, France

Müller-Lissner S., Abteilung für Innere Medizin, Krankenhaus Weissensee, Schönstr. 85-91, D - 13086 Berlin, Germany.

Pascaud X., Institut de Recherche Jouveinal, 3-9, rue de la Loge, 94265 Fresnes Cedex, France.

Read N.W., Centre for Human Nutrition, Northern General Hospital, Herries Road, Sheffield, UK.

Rivière P.J.M., Institut de Recherche Jouveinal, 3-9, rue de la Loge, 94265 Fresnes Cedex, France.

Scherrer B., Institut de Recherche Jouveinal, 3-9, rue de la Loge, 94265 Fresnes Cedex, France.

Schwizer W., Policlinique Médicale Universitaire, 19, rue César-Roux, 1005 Lausanne, Switzerland.

Sengupta J.N., Department of Pharmacology, College of Medicine, University of Iowa, Iowa City, IA 52242, USA.

Sensitive gastrointestinal disorders. J.P. Galmiche, B. Fraitag.
John Libbey Eurotext, Paris © 1995, pp. 1-2

Introduction

E. CORAZZIARI

*II Clinica Medica, Policlinico Umberto I, Università degli studi La Sapienza,
Cattedra di Gastroenterologia, 00161 Roma Italia.*

The proceedings of this book put an end to a research period of over thirty years, which has interpreted functional gastrointestinal (GI) disorders as the outcome of altered motor control and activity, and set the stage for a period which will offer increasing consideration to the role of visceral afference and sensitivity in these disturbances.

It is not surprising that deranged bowel habits in the « irritable colon syndrome », or immediate postprandial satiety and epigastric distension in endoscopy-negative dyspepsia, have been interpreted as an expression of altered motor activity, respectively, of the large bowel and the stomach. More unexpected, and increasingly frustrating for the clinicians, has been the accumulating evidence that, parallel to the demonstrations of altered GI motor activity in functional GI disorders, there could be little relationship between the motor derangements and the patients' complaints. Thus, some functional GI disorders, such as those affecting the sphincter of Oddi, the oro-pharynx, the pelvic floor, and the anal sphincters, are closely associated with disturbances in visceral or somatic motor function. In other functional disorders presenting with chronic or recurrent pain, such as esophageal chest pain, dyspepsia and irritable bowel syndrome, motor abnormalities may be found but are not as closely linked to symptoms as the disturbances in visceral sensations. Finally, patients with functional abdominal pain and bloating syndromes present disturbances in visceral sensations and/or behaviour and little or no motor abnormalities. At the same time, it has been recognized that drugs effective on GI motility and capable of reverting motor dysfunction could have a limited role on the patients' symptoms.

All this accumulating knowledge has led to the theory that functional GI disorders result from the multifactorial interchange played by altered GI motor, sensory and central nervous system activity through the brain-gut afferent and efferent connections and, within the gut, between the enteric nervous system and the sensory-motor function.

These proceedings offer an overview of the available evidence played by deranged visceral afference and sensitivity in the pathogenesis of functional GI disorders presenting with chronic or recurrent abdominal pain. Potentially useful for future application are the descriptions of new methods used to assess and measure the disturbances of visceral afference and sensitivity in functional dyspepsia and irritable bowel syndrome. Being linked to the development of a new drug, which acts on visceral afference, these proceedings offer an overview of the subtypes of opioid receptors and fully cover the role of peripheral kappa opioid receptors in the modulation of afference and visceral sensitivity. Although not a comprehensive review of the kappa opioid agonists, this book, published with so little delay from the conference held in Versailles, indeed offers an extensive description of the action of fedotozine on the visceral afferent fibers and of its effect on gastric and intestinal nociception. Evidence of the peripheral action of fedotozine, as well as its satisfactory safety profile, are reported in several studies. Finally the conference has been the occasion to present the promising results of the pilot clinical studies and of the first, some of which still ongoing, controlled clinical trials on the efficacy of fedotozine in the treatment of functional GI disorders.

First session

Functional dyspepsia and irritable bowel syndrome. Growing evidence supporting sensitive disturbances

Sensitive gastrointestinal disorders. J.P. Galmiche, B. Fraitag.
John Libbey Eurotext, Paris © 1995, pp. 5-9

1

Overview of factors involved in functional disorders of the gastrointestinal tract

S. MÜLLER-LISSNER

Abteilung für Innere Medizin, Krankenhaus Weissensee, Berlin, Germany.

Definitions and general considerations

Irritable bowel syndrome (IBS) has recently been defined as "a functional bowel disorder in which abdominal pain is associated with defaecation or a change in bowel habit, and with features of disordered defaecation and with distension", where "functional" means "not explained by structural or biochemical abnormalities" [1]. Problems with this definition and similar ones are twofold. First, "IBS" is suggested to be a single disease entity ("... a functional bowel disorder ..."). Second, thorough investigation of patients with "IBS" - at present or after further research - may detect a structural or biochemical abnormality. Thus, a patient with an hitherto functional disorder would afterwards suffer from an organic disease. In the following, a functional disorder of the lower gastrointestinal (GI) tract is assumed when the patient complains of chronically disturbed defaecation, preferably in association with abdominal complaints such as pain or distension, and if physical examination, laboratory investigations for neoplastic, infectious and inflammatory causes, abdominal ultrasound, and colonoscopy do not reveal a cause.

The term dyspepsia should be used to describe symptoms which are experienced in the upper abdomen and are referred by the attending physician to the upper GI tract including biliary system, liver, and pancreas. Hence, symptoms such as jaundice, gastrointestinal bleeding, acid regurgitation and dysphagia do not belong to dyspepsia. Dyspepsia of more than a couple of weeks duration is called chronic dyspepsia. If the cause of dyspepsia remains obscure after physical examination, laboratory investigations for neoplastic, infectious and inflammatory causes, abdominal ultrasound, and upper GI endoscopy, it may be called functional (or idiopathic, or essential) dyspepsia. (FD) Synonyma such as gastritis and non-ulcer dyspepsia (NUD) are less well suited since gastritis is a histological diagnosis and is probably asymptomatic, and since the term NUD would also include, *e.g.,* gastric or pancreatic cancer.

According to the above definitions, disaccharidase deficiency is classified as a functional disorder. Here at last some readers will disagree. But what is the difference between a patient who complains of distension, flatulence, and loose stools who benefits from a lactose free diet and another with the same symptoms who benefits from omitting whole grain products ?

Further, in patients with slow colonic transit constipation, abnormalities of the enteric nervous system have been found. Should these patients therefore be classified as suffering from organic colonic disease ? And what about patients with disordered defaecation due to a rectocele or an intussusception A morphological method (defaecography) shows the abnormality but only when the function (defaecation) is activated. Obviously also the terms "functional" (if it has something to do with function) and "organic" are not very well chosen because organic diseases affect function as well. However, these terms are widely used and it would be nearly impossible to change them. The probably most convincing difference between disorders labelled "organic" and ''functional'' is that the former usually harbours the danger of deterioration, complications, or serious outcome, *i.e.* a bad prognosis if untreated whereas the latter usually does not. That is the reason why our above definition of functional disease includes a specification of a minimal diagnostic programme and thereby an operational definition of organic disease (Figure 1).

What is behind dyspepsia ?

Around 5% of the population seek medical advice for dyspeptic symptoms [2]. In less than half of these, an organic cause for the symptoms such as a peptic ulcer or carcinoma can be found. In about half of the remaining patients, a functional cause for the symptoms may be identified with available methodology [3] (Table I). The most frequent cause of FD and dyspepsia in general probably is gastro-oesophageal reflux (with or without erosive oesophagitis) with "atypical" - namely epigastric - symptoms. The second frequent cause is gastrointestinal hypomotility.

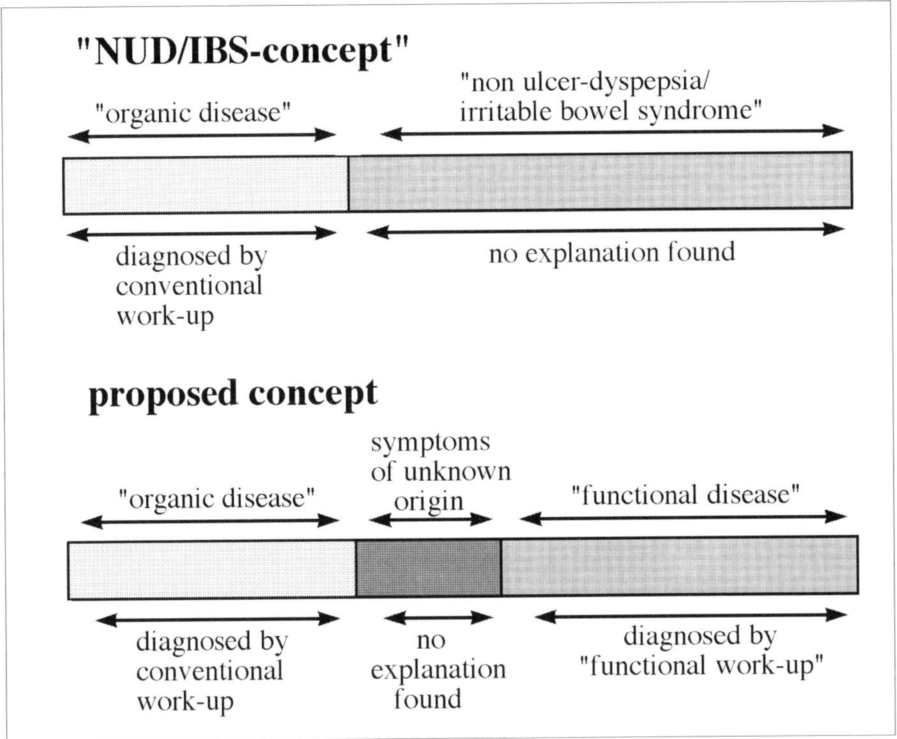

Figure 1. Graphic representation of the classical "non-ulcer dyspepsia / irritable bowel syndrome"-concept and the proposed concept where the classification of a disorder as organic or functional is mainly based on the type of the diagnostic procedure applied. "Conventional work-up" means physical examination, laboratory investigations for neoplastic, infectious and inflammatory causes, abdominal ultrasound, and upper GI endoscopy or colonoscopy, respectively. "Functional work-up" means tests such as long-term oesophageal pH monitoring, manometry, or test treatment.

Table I. Possible findings in patients with symptoms considered characteristic for "functional dyspepsia" when work-up including upper gastrointestinal endoscopy was negative.

- Gastro-oesophageal reflux disease

- Gastric hypomotility

- Small intestinal hypomotility ("pseudo-obstruction")

- Low threshold for gastric distension

- Sphincter of Oddi dyskinesia

- Intolerance for sugars (lactose, fructose, sorbitol)

- Side effects of drugs and other compounds

What is behind the irritable bowel syndrome ?

There is a whole body of abnormalities which may be found in patients suffering from IBS. These disorders may be well known for quite a long time (*e.g.*, lactase deficiency) or identified more recently (*e.g.*, slow colonic transit, obstructed defaecation) (Table II).

Table II. Possible findings in patients with symptoms considered characteristic for the irritable bowel syndrome when work-up including colonoscopy was negative.

- Fibre deficiency of diet

- Intolerance for sugars (lactose, fructose, sorbitol)

- Low threshold for distension of rectosigmoid colon

- Intolerance for dietary fibre

- Slow colonic transit (despite high fibre diet)

- Side effects of drugs and other compounds

- Functional outlet obstruction (internal prolapse, rectocele, anismus, Hirschsprung's disease)

Disordered function : the cause of symptoms ?

Tables I and II are likely to be incomplete. Further studies may reveal other pathophysiological entities. In addition, two minor abnormalities may produce symptoms only when occurring together, *e.g.*, a certain amount of disaccharide malabsorption may only become symptomatic if the threshold for perception is abnormally low [4]. And, of course, minor symptoms may only become a medical problem if the patient consults a doctor, *e.g.*, as a consequence of learned illness behaviour [5]. It should be stressed that an abnormality found in a test is not necessarily the cause of the symptoms. If there is a specific therapeutic option, its success may prove causality. For surgical procedures, however, such as fundoplication or correction of a rectocele, the treatment is irreversible and should therefore only be applied if the success can be predicted with a reasonable likelihood. The demand for causality between a demonstrated abnormality and symptoms is much more strict than in organic diseases. If one finds carcinoma upon colonoscopy which was performed for diarrhoea, one would not wonder whether the tumour is the cause of diarrhoea or not, since there is a prognostic, and not only a symptomatic aim of treatment in nearly every organic disease (*see* above).

References

1. Thompson WG, Creed F, Drossman DA, Heaton KW, Mazzacca G. Functional bowel disease and functional abdominal pain. *Gastroenterol Int* 1992 ; 5 : 75-91.
2. Jones RH, Lydeard SE, Hobbs FDR, Kenkre JE, Williams EI, Jones SJ, Repper JA, Caldow JL, Dunwoodie WMB, Bottomley JM. Dyspepsia in England and Scotland. *Gut* 1990 ; 31 : 401-15.
3. Klauser AG, Voderholzer W, Knesewitsch AP, Schindlbeck NE, Müller-Lissner SA. What is behind dyspepsia ? *Dig Dis Sci* 1993 ; 38 : 147-54.
4. Fernandez-Benarez F, Esteve-Pardo M, de Leon R, Humbert P, Carbe E, Llovet JM, Gassull MA. Sugar malabsorption in functional bowel disease: clinical implications. *Am J Gastroenterol* 1993 ; 88 : 2044-50.
5. Whitehead WE, Winget C, Fedoravicius AS, Wooley S, Blackwell B. Learned illness behaviour in patients with irritable bowel syndrome and peptic ulcer. *Dig Dis Sci* 1982 ; 27 : 202-8.

Sensitive gastrointestinal disorders. J.P. Galmiche, B. Fraitag.
John Libbey Eurotext, Paris © 1995, pp. 11-14

2

Altered sensory perception as a basis for symptom generation in functional bowel disorders

S.M. COLLINS

Intestinal Diseases Research Unit, McMaster University, Hamilton, Ontario, Canada.

Conceptually, functional bowel disorders (FBD) embrace a wide variety of clinical conditions that range from non-cardiac chest pain (of oesophageal origin), to functional dyspepsia (FD) and irritable bowel syndrome (IBS).

Traditionally, the gastrointestinal features of these conditions have been considered to be manifestations of abnormal motility, reflecting a disorder of smooth muscle or enteric nerves or both. There has, however, been no robust demonstration of a primary abnormality of smooth muscle, despite initial claims of a 3 cycle per minute dominant slow wave frequency of myoelectrical activity in the colon of patients with IBS. In non-ulcer dyspepsia (NUD), abnormalities of gastric motility (antral hypomotility) have been found in about only a half of cases studied. While some have been able to report a correlation between abnormal motor patterns and symptoms [1], the majority of studies have not found this to be robust. Consequently, attention has turned to alternative explanations of symptoms in FBD.

It has long been known that patients with IBS have been intolerant to balloon distension of the rectum [2], suggesting a possible mechanism for abdominal pain through increased visceral sensitivity [3]. However, because such patients frequently express non-gastrointestinal symptoms, and are known to seek medical attention more frequently than others [4], these findings were interpreted to reflect a generalized intolerance of the patient to discomfort, rather than a manifestation of altered sensory perception in the gut.

This notion was examined in a study by Cook *et al.* [5], in which they measured values for threshold perception and maximum tolerance of pain inflicted on the forearm of IBS patients by electric shock. That study used healthy subjects as negative controls and a cohort of age and sex-matched patients with chronic pain due to Crohn's disease. The results were counter-intuitive in that the IBS patients exhibited a higher value for threshold and maximum tolerance than the healthy subjects, and their profile was similar to that observed in the Crohn's disease patients. These findings were interpreted to indicate that the gut was the likely source of pain in these patients.

Pain is the commonest symptom in FBD and yet treatment is far from satisfactory. Drugs aimed at relieving pain by reducing muscle contraction (anti-spasmodics) have enjoyed limited success as central analgesics which run a risk of psychological dependence among these patients in particular. The need for a new mode of treating pain in this group is long overdue.

Work primarily performed in other systems has generated sufficient data upon which to base a hypothesis for the development of visceral hyperalgesia potentially applicable to FBD [6].

Sensations in the gut are received initially by chemo- or mechano-receptors and generate impulses in afferent sensory fibres. These may be divided into low-threshold A-delta fibres that are rapidly adapting and encode mainly phasic stimuli and C fibres that are slowly adapting and encode tonic stimuli. There is a significant population of C fibres that remain silent under normal conditions but which may become activated following local inflammation or irritation. Works done mainly in the urinary bladder [7] have shown that experimental cystitis causes the recruitment of such fibres. The increased input of afferent activity converges on the second order neuron in the dorsal horn of the spinal cord, which then undergoes plastic change with resulting lower thresholds and increased maximum responses for a given input.The sensitized second order neuron provides increased input to higher centres, resulting in the perception of pain or other noxious sensations. These changes in the second order neuron long outlast the sensitizing events in the periphery, thereby giving rise to a peripheral mechanism for visceral hyperalgesia. (For review, also *see* [6].)

The strategically important second order neuron is also subject to facilitatory or inhibitory modulation from higher centres *via* spinal pathways. The second order neuron may be modulated directly through these descending pathways to achieve a state of sensitization, either through reduced descending inhibition, or conversely through increased descending facilitation. Thus, a pathway of visceral hyperalgesia exists whereby central neural actions may be an initiating factor. The relative contributions of peripheral and central mechanisms in the development of visceral hyperalgesia in FBD is unknown ; since this is likely to be a mechanistically heterogeneous clinical entity, defined principally by its clinical expression, it is likely that both pathways are relevant.

In considering the feasibility of applying current concepts of visceral hyperalgesia to the topic of FBD, one must first consider putative pathogenetic pathways in these disorders. These disorders are heterogeneous not only in terms of their clinical presentation but also in terms of their pathogenesis, which is also likely to be multifactorial. Traditionally emphasis has been placed on behavioural factors, with the recognition that these patients, as a group, tend to exhibit high scores for anxiety and depression. Stress has also been implicated in the expression of these disorders, as has sleep deprivation.

Mental, but not physical, stress has been shown to cause increased discomfort on balloon distension of the rectum in healthy subjects [8]. Similarly, sleep deprivation [9] in healthy volunteers produced IBS-like symptoms as well as intolerance to balloon distension of the rectum. These observations suggest the feasibility of a centrally induced visceral hyperalgesic state in FBD.

Approximately 33% of irritable bowel is believed to occur following an enteric infection [10] and it has recently been shown that approximately 30% of patients experiencing an episode of salmonella gastroenteritis developed IBS-like symptoms after three months. These patients also exhibited reduced tolerance to balloon distension [11]. This observation suggests that peripheral mechanisms leading to hyperalgesia may be operative in some patients with FBD.

Considering that inflammation is the cardinal process that leads to hyperalgesia in several systems, it seems reasonable to consider the evidence supporting an inflammatory basis at least in some patients with FBD.

Several studies have shown increased numbers of inflammatory cells in the mucosa, lamina propria or muscularis externa of patients with FD (stomach) or IBS (ileum and colon), and this has been recently reviewed [12]. We have preliminary data showing increased expression of interleukin-1β and MCH II mRNA in colonic mucosal biopsy specimens from patients with diarrhoea predominant IBS [13]. *In vitro* studies have shown, at least in animals, that IL-1β induces an increase in substance P in nerves in the gut, and we speculate that this may influence pain perception.

In summary, therefore, there is a growing awareness of increased sensory perception, or visceral hyperalgesia, as a basis for pain in FBD. Although our understanding of the precise mechanisms leading to a chronic state of hyperalgesia in these conditions is in its infancy, there is sufficient evidence to suggest that both peripheral and central mechanisms may play a role. The former is important as it may lend itself to pharmacomodulation without involving central nervous system directly, and thereby avoiding many of the constraints imposed on using centrally acting analgesics in these disorders. Kappa opiates are known to attenuate sensory perception in the periphery and the availability of fedotozine, a kappa ligand, constitutes an exciting new prospect in the management of this common but difficult category of disorders.

References

1. Kellow JE, Eckersley G, Jones MP. Enhanced perception of physiological intestinal motility in the irritable bowel syndrome. *Gastroenterology* 1991 ; 101 :1621-7.
2. Whitehead WE, Holtkotter B, Enck P, Hoelzl R, Holmes KD, Anthony J, *et al.* Tolerance for rectosigmoid distension in irritable bowel syndrome. *Gastroenterology* 1990 ; 98 : 1187-92.
3. Bradette M, Delvaux M, Staumont G, Fioramonti J, Bueno L, Frexinos J. Evaluation of colonic sensory thresholds in IBS patients using a barostat. Definition of optimal conditions and comparison with healthy subjects. *Dig Dis Sci* 1994 ; 39 : 449-57.
4. Whitehead WE, Crowell MD. Psychologic considerations in the irritable bowel syndrome. *Gastroenterol Clin North Am* 1991 ; 20 : 249-67.
5. Cook IJ, van Eeden A, Collins SM. Patients with irritable bowel syndrome have greater pain tolerance than normal subjects. *Gastroenterology* 1987 ; 93 : 727-33.
6. Mayer EA, Gebhart GF. Basic and clinical aspects of visceral hyperalgesia. *Gastroenterology* 1994 ; 107 : 271-93.
7. McMahon S, Koltzenburg M. The changing role of primary afferent neurons in pain. *Pain* 1990 ; 43 : 269-72.
8. Erckenbrecht J.F. Noise and intestinal motor alterations. In : Bueno L, Collins SM, Junien JL, eds. *Stress and digestive motility*. London, Paris : John Libbey Co, 1989 : 93-6.
9. Bergin AJ, Read NW. The effects of sleep deprivation on rectal sensitivity in healthy volunteers. *Eur J Gastroenterol Hepatol* 1993 ; 5 : 527-32.
10. Chaudhary NA, Truelove SC. The irritable bowel syndrome. *Q J Med* 1962 ; 31 : 307-22.
11. Bergin AJ, Donnelly TC, McKendrick MW, Read NW. Changes in anorectal function in persistent bowel disturbance following salmonella gastroenteritis. *Eur J Gastroenterol Hepatol* 1993 ; 5 : 617-20.
12. Collins SM. Is the irritable gut an inflamed gut ? *Scand J Gastroenterol* 1992 ; 192 (Suppl.) : 102-5.
13. Collins SM, Hurst SM, Main C, Stanley E, Khan L, Blennerhassett P, *et al.* Effect of inflammation of enteric nerves. Cytokine-induced changes in neurotransmitter content and release. *Ann NY Acad Sci* 1992 ; 664 : 415-24.

Sensitive gastrointestinal disorders. J.P. Galmiche, B. Fraitag.
John Libbey Eurotext, Paris © 1995, pp. 15-21

3

Viscero-perception

F. AZPIROZ

Digestive System Research Unit, Hospital General Vall d'Hebron, Autonomous University of Barcelona, Spain.

In normal conditions, physiological *stimuli* in the gut induce regulatory reflexes, so that the digestive process evolves unperceived. For instance, the nutrient composition of chyme along the small intestine regulates the contraction of the stomach, and hence, the amount of nutrients delivered into the small intestine. In dogs, with an isolated loop of small intestine, we used a barostat to monitor gastric tone (Figure 1). The barostat is a feedback mechanism that maintains a low and constant pressure level within an intragastric bag, and measures the volume required to maintain this pressure level [1, 2]. Infusion of a fat solution into the intestine induced a gastric relaxation, and when the infusion was stopped, gastric tone recovered [3].

In humans, duodenal distension produces a gastric relaxatory response, which is very similar to that produced by intestinal nutrients (Figure 2). However, this kind of stimulus also produces perception [4]. The most frequent symptoms induced by intestinal distension are abdominal pressure, fullness and bloating. Interestingly, the same kind of symptoms can be elicited by distension of different parts of the gut, from the stomach down to the jejunum [5-7]. Most patients with functional disorders complain of similar sensations ; for instance, dyspeptic patients complain of abdominal pressure or fullness after meals [5]. However, what does really produce the symptoms ? Are symptoms produced by an excessive contraction of the stomach and gastric hypertension or are they produced by a hypotonic elongation of the stomach. We addressed this question in a series of studies as follows [8]. Basically, there are two methods to produce distension of the gut. We can either inject fixed volumes of air within an intraluminal bag and measure the changes in intraluminal pressure, or we can

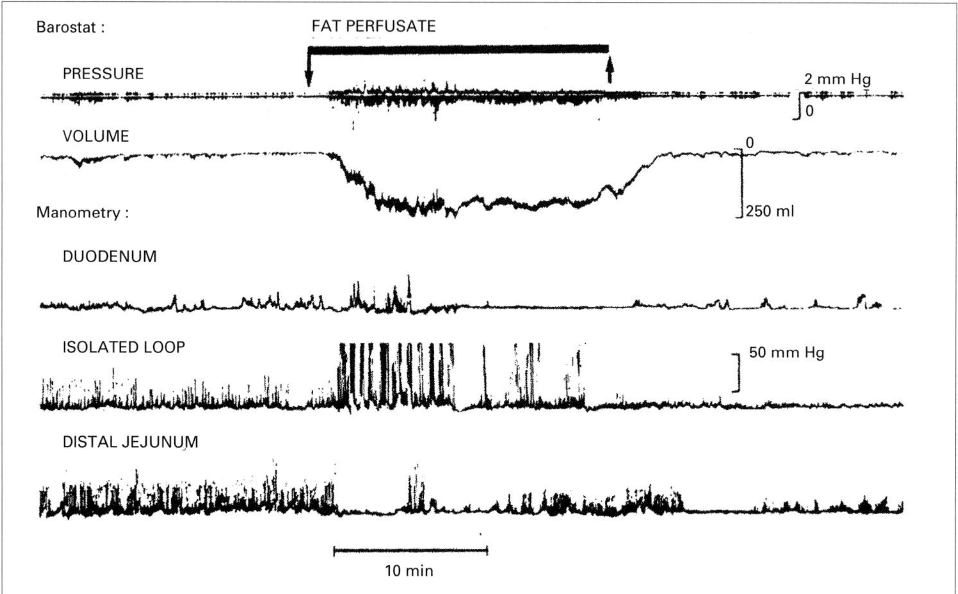

Figure 1. Gastric tone monitored by gastric barostat and intestinal motility monitored by manometry in a conscious dog with an isolated loop of intestine. Fat perfusion into the isolated loop produced a reflex gastric relaxation (barostat volume enlarged at constant pressure) and stimulated motility in the isolated loop.

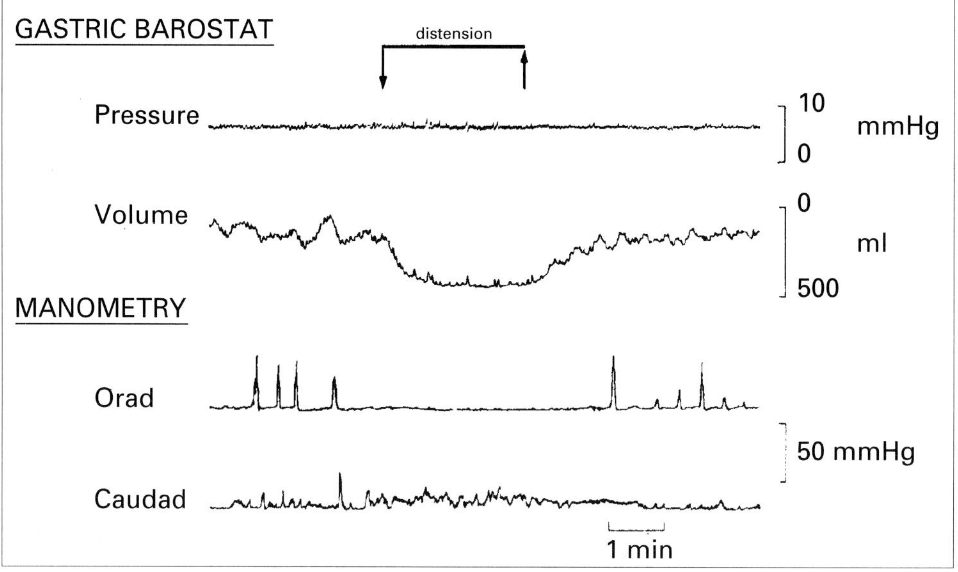

Figure 2. Gastric tone monitored by gastric barostat and phasic motility monitored by manometry orad and caudad to a duodenal balloon in a healthy subject. Duodenal balloon distension produced a reflex gastric relaxation. From [4].

use a barostat that maintains a fixed pressure level and measures the volume changes. In a group of healthy subjects, we used these two techniques. We compared the responses using volumetric and barostat distensions, when the stomach was contracted during basal conditions and when the stomach was relaxed by glucagon. We used a graded questionnaire to quantify the intensity of the symptoms by a perception score. We found that, at the same pressure levels, the intragastric volumes and perception scores were much greater when the stomach was relaxed. By contrast, at the same distending volumes, the intragastric pressures and perception scores were much smaller when the stomach was relaxed. When we maintain a constant intragastric pressure, the stomach can detect differences in intragastric volume, and when we maintain a constant intragastric volume, the stomach is able to detect differences in intragastric pressure. These data suggest that there should be two kinds of receptors signalling the distension of the stomach : *i.e.* (1) "in parallel" elongation receptors that will behave as volume receptors ; and (2) "in series" tension receptors that will detect changes in intragastric pressure. Following this model, symptoms can be produced either by isometric contraction of the stomach due to excessive tension, or symptoms can be produced by isotonic relaxation due to an excessive elongation of the gut wall.

There are a variety of mechanisms, between the gut and the brain, that modulate the sensory imput at different levels of the afferent path, and thus regulate the intensity of perception of gut *stimuli.*

Inflation of an intestinal balloon in healthy subjects induces stimulus-related perception. Simultaneous inflation of a second balloon nearby with a small volume that is just perceived produces a shift of the stimulus response curve to the left : volumes that are well tolerated alone produce discomfort when a small stimulus is simultaneously applied [9]. Finally, the gut responds to simultaneous stimulation by a phenomenon of spatial summation.

What happens if a somatic stimulus is combined with a visceral stimulus ? In a group of healthy subjects, we used a gastric barostat to produce gastric distension, and an intestinal barostat to produce duodenal distension. We performed the distensions either alone or with simultaneous application of transcutaneous electrical nerve stimulation on the hand. Somatic *stimuli* increased the tolerance both to gastric distension and to duodenal distension [10]. In contrast to visceral *stimuli* which produce a phenomenon of summation, here we have a phenomenon of desensitization. Possibly, this kind of mechanism may be activated by acupuncture.

The sympathetic nervous system also participates in the regulation of perception. Lower body negative pressure (LBNP) is a very elegant method to produce activation of the sympathetic nervous system. The subjects are placed within a rigid box which is hermetically closed ; LBNP is produced by air suction up to a level of -40 mmHg. LBNP produces a venous pooling that activates the sympathetic nervous system by a peripheral mechanism without modifying vagal activity. In a group of healthy subjects, we measured the perception of the same *stimuli,* applied during sham LBNP (at atmospheric pressure) and during active LBNP (at -40 mmHg). Activation of the sympathetic nervous system by LBNP significantly increased perception of duodenal distension. However, sympathetic activation did not modify perception of somatic *stimuli*, such as transcutaneous electrical nerve stimulation applied on the hand [11]. This is very interesting because it is exactly what we find in some functional patients, which have hypersensitivity to gut *stimuli*, but normal sensitivity to somatic *stimuli*. Furthermore, this kind of mechanism might participate in the pathogenesis of the irritable bowel syndrome (IBS), because some recent data have shown that IBS patients have increased sympathetic activity.

On top of all the regulatory mechanisms, perception is finally modulated by cognitive processes at the level of the brain cortex. In a very carefully designed experiment, we compared perception of intestinal *stimuli* applied during mental attention by anticipatory knowledge and during mental distraction by simple calculations. These studies showed that mental attention increases perception of gut distension [12].

Intestinal distension produces perception but also produces visceral reflexes. Are these two responses related to each other or are they independent ? If we produce low level distension of the duodenum, we induce a reflex relaxation of the stomach without perception at all. Therefore, the enterogastric reflex relaxation is independent of perception. If we produce distension of the duodenum at higher levels, both responses will be obtained. Distension of the jejunum produces the same type and the same intensity of perception as that of the duodenum, but without any reflex response of the stomach. Therefore, perception is also independent of the reflex response [13]. These data suggest that these two responses are probably produced by specific mechanisms. Consequently, being independent, they may also be independently altered in some patients. In a specific group of dyspeptic patients with the "bloating syndrome", we studied the effect of gastric and duodenal distensions using two separate barostats. We found that dyspeptic patients had a reduced tolerance to gastric distension, with a completely normal sensitivity of the duodenum. However, these patients had an impaired gastric relaxation in response to duodenal distension [5]. Therefore dyspeptic patients may have a gastric hypersensitivity, but also an associated gastric hyporeactivity.

Using distending *stimuli* in the gut, abnormalities can be detected in functional patients. However, distension of the gut produces perception *via* activation of mechano-receptors in the gut wall, and we cannot determine the level of the dysfunction. For that purpose, we have developed an alternative method of sensory testing, namely, transmucosal electrical nerve stimulation [14]. Electrical stimulation is applied *via* a bipolar electrode mounted over an intestinal tube (Figure 3). Transmucosal electrical nerve stimulation produces the same symptoms as intestinal distension, such as colicky sensation, pressure fullness or sharp sensation. Only less than one third of electrical *stimuli* are perceived as paresthesia or flutter-like sensation. Comparison of the perception score at different intensities of electrical stimulation and at different distending volumes showed that transmucosal electrical nerve stimulation and

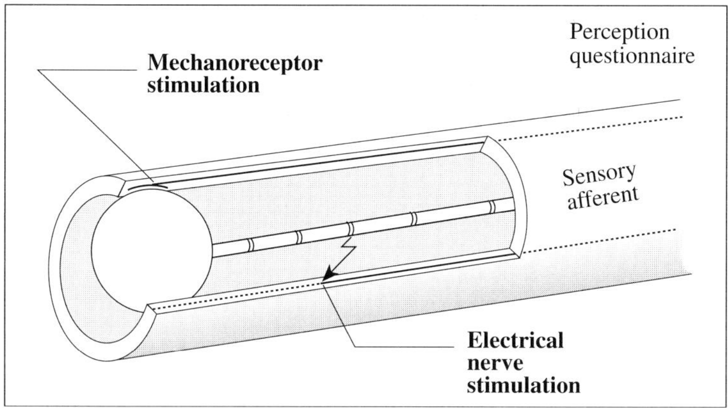

Figure 3. Intestinal distension activates sensory afferents *via* mechanoreceptor stimulation, whereas transmucosal electrical nerve stimulation does not rely on any specific receptor. From [14].

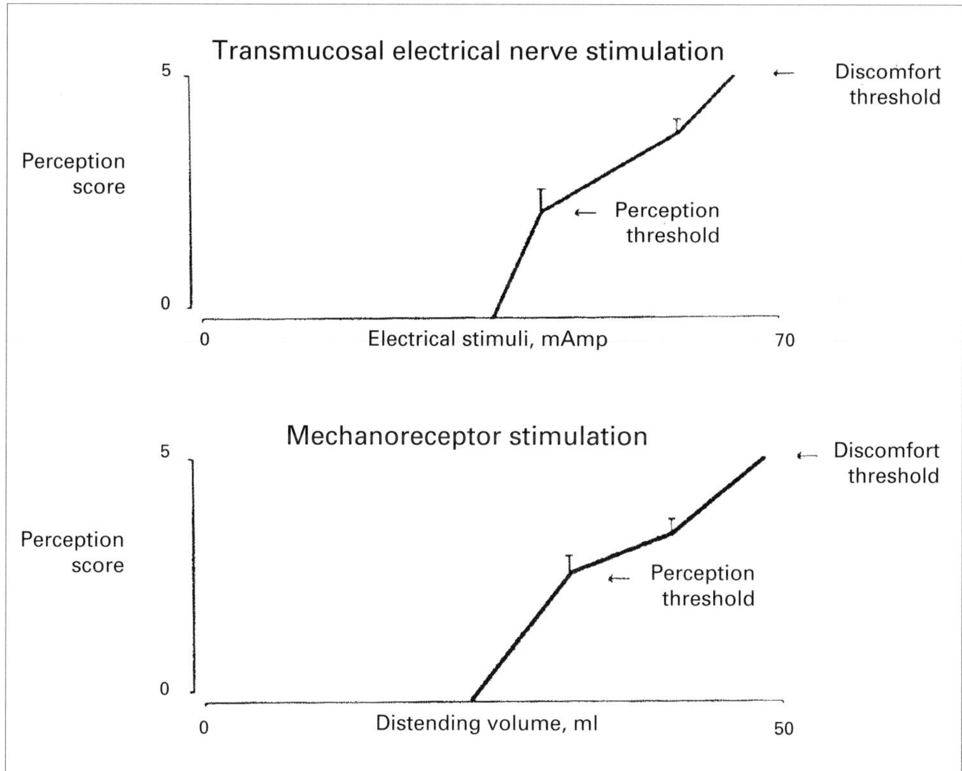

Figure 4. Perception score in response to transmucosal electrical nerve stimulation and mechanoreceptor stimulation in human. Both produce similar stimulus-related perception.

mechanical stimulation produce very similar stimulus-related perception from the perception threshold up to the threshold for discomfort (Figure 4).

We applied this technique to study a group of patients with IBS. It is well established that patients with IBS have a hypersensitivity of the colon and the rectum.We performed mechanoreceptor stimulation by balloon distension and transmucosal electrical nerve stimulation of the jejunum in patients with IBS and in healthy controls. We found that IBS patients perceived and tolerated smaller intestinal volumes than healthy controls. However, the sensitivity to transmucosal electrical nerve stimulation was similar both in patients and in healthy subjects suggesting a selective alteration of mechanosensitive pathways [15].

In summary, physiological *stimuli* in the gut normally produce reflex responses to regulate the digestive process. In certain conditions, gut *stimuli* may produce perception of symptoms. Both the reflex responses and perception are modulated by a variety of mechanisms along the brain gut axis. Some patients with functional disorders may have a hypersensitivity of the gut and physiological *stimuli* may induce symptoms. What seems interesting is that different types of functional disorders may share a common pathophysiological mechanism and the specific clinical presentation may depend on the topography of the dysfunction.

References

1. Azpiroz F, Malagelada JR. Physiologic variations in canine gastric tone measured by an electronic barostat. *Am J Physiol* 1985 ; 248 : G229-37.
2. Azpiroz F, Malagelada JR. Gastric tone measured by an electronic barostat in health and postsurgical gastroparesis. *Gastroenterology* 1987 ; 92 : 934-43.
3. Azpiroz F, Malagelada JR. Intestinal control of gastric tone. *Am J Physiol* 1985.; 249 : G501-9.
4. Azpiroz F, Malagelada JR. Perception and reflex relaxation of the stomach in response to gut distension. *Gastroenterology* 1990 ; 98 : 1193-8.
5. Coffin B, Azpiroz F, Guarner F, Malagelada JR. Selective gastric hypersensitivity and reflex hyporeactivity in functional dyspepsia. *Gastroenterology* 1994 ; 107 : 1345-51.
6. Rouillon JM, Azpiroz F, Malagelada JR. Reflex changes in intestinal tone: relationship to perception. *Am J Physiol* 1991 ; 261 : G280-6.
7. Rouillon JM, Azpiroz F, Malagelada JR. Sensorial in intestino-intestinal reflex pathways in the human jejunum. *Gastroenterology* 1991 ; 101 : 1606-12.
8. Notivol R, Coffin B, Azpiroz F, Mearin F, Serra J, Malagelada JR. Gastric tone determines the sensitivity of the stomach to distension. *Gastroenterology* 1995 ; 108 : 330-6.
9. Serra J, Azpiroz F, Malagelada JR. Temporo-spatial modulation of perception and reflex responses to intestinal *stimuli* in humans. *Gastroenterology* 1994 ; 106 : A565.
10. Coffin B, Azpiroz F, Malagelada JR. Somatic stimulation reduces perception of gut distension. *Gastroenterology* 1994 ; 107 : 1636-42.
11. Iovino P, Azpiroz F, Domingo E, Malagelada JR.The sympathetic nervous system modulates perception and reflex responses to gut distension in humans. *Gastroenterology* 1995 ; 108 : 680-6.
12. Accarino AM, Azpiroz F, Malagelada JR. Focusing attention at the gut : effects on viscero-visceral reflexes and perception. *Gastroenterology* 1993 ; 104 : A468.

13. Azpiroz F, Malagelada JR. Isobaric intestinal distension in humans: sensorial relay and reflex gastric relaxation. *Am J Physiol* 1990 ; 258 : G202-7.
14. Accarino AM, Azpiroz F, Malagelada JR. Symptomatic responses to stimulation of sensory pathways in the jejunum. *Am J Physiol* 1992 ; 263 : G673-7.
15. Accarino AM, Azpiroz F, Malagelada JR. Selective dysfunction of mechanosensitive intestinal afferents in the irritable bowel syndrome. *Gastroenterology* 1995 ; 108 : 636-43.

Sensitive gastrointestinal disorders. J.P. Galmiche, B. Fraitag.
John Libbey Eurotext, Paris © 1995, pp. 23-30

4

Role of peripheral kappa receptors in the modulation of pain

J.L. JUNIEN

Institut de Recherche Jouveinal, Fresnes, France.

Opioid receptors are classified as µ-, δ- and κ-receptors. All these receptors have been cloned, and so far there is only one type of clones which has been expressed for each, but binding experiments have provided the evidence that some subtypes do exist for all these receptors : in the case of the κ- receptor, they are named κ-1a,b, κ-2 and κ-3. All the µ-, δ- and κ-receptors are linked to a G-protein and the second messenger systems are the adenylcyclase system, calcium and potassium channels. Specific agonists are compounds from the arylacetamide series as U-50,488H and PD-117,302. They are more or less selective to the κ-1 receptors : fedotozine is selective for the κ-1a, bremazocine for κ-1, κ-2 and it has some affinity for µ-receptors also.Dynorphins are the endogenous ligands for κ-receptors. Selective antagonists are nor-binaltorphimine (nor-BN)I, which is a κ-1 and κ-2 selective antagonist, naloxone which is a selective antagonist for µ- receptors at low doses, but displays a universal blocking effect for any of these receptors when used at higher doses.

What are the evidences for a peripheral site of action of opioids in pain ? This has been largely documented for many years now by different groups [1-3]. These groups have essentially used the same techniques. They have tested the effect of a low amount of opioids injected either systemically or at the site where the pain occurs. This very low amount of drug was not able to produce systemic activity but antinociception after local administration. Figure 1 shows an experiment done by Stein *et al.* [4]. They used a classical model of pain where Freund's adjuvant is injected in the paw of the rat. The animals are tested five days later and the effect of drugs can be investigated by measuring the paw pressure threshold where the animal withdraws his paw. A low dose (50 µg) of the κ-agonist U-50,488H is injected in the paw. There is an antinociceptive

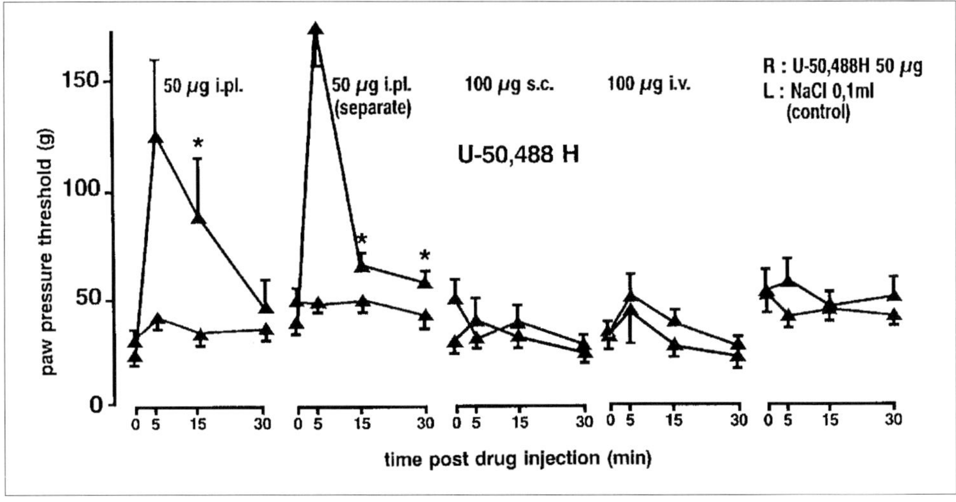

Figure 1. Paw pressure threshold elevation after intraplantar injection of low dose U-50,488H (50µg) not active systemically. (Reprinted with kind permission from [5].)

response which corresponds to an elevation of the paw pressure threshold. This effect is seen in the inflamed paw, but not observed in the normal paw. These results were found in two different groups of animals. In one group the same animals were tested at different times and, in the other one, different animals were tested at different times to avoid any learning interference. Even with a double dose of U-50,488H injected by s.c. or by i.v. route, no antinociceptive response was observed. These results indicate clearly that one can have an antinociceptive effect of the κ-agonist U-50,488H when it is injected locally, at a non-systemic dose, and also show that a better response is occurring at the site which is already inflamed.

What is the mode of action of opioid ligands ? It has been shown by many groups that opioid receptors are present in the sensory nerves [5,6]. For instance, two kinds of experiments have been done which support this. Immuno-staining with a mouse monoclonal antibody for the µ- and δ-receptors has been reported by Hassan *et al.* [5]. No antibodies for the κ-receptors were available. Cutaneous nerves are labelled with this mouse antibody. There is a clear increase in the labelling with these monoclonal antibodies in animals pretreated with Freund's adjuvant. Sengupta and Gebhart [7] have used another approach. The sciatic nerve has been ligatured downstream the dorsal root ganglion. They have examined two different segments, above the ligature in P1 and P2 to the dorsal root ganglion, and D1 and D2 to the peripheral endings (Figure 2). These two segments were taken away, and the binding was determined using cold ligands and ^{3}H bremazocine for labelling the µ- and the κ-receptors. The open bar corresponds to the normal condition and the black bar corresponds to nerves taken from animals having already an inflammation. µ-opioid binding is largely increased in P1 and D1, and the same occurs with the κ-binding on the proximal site close to the ligature, but not much

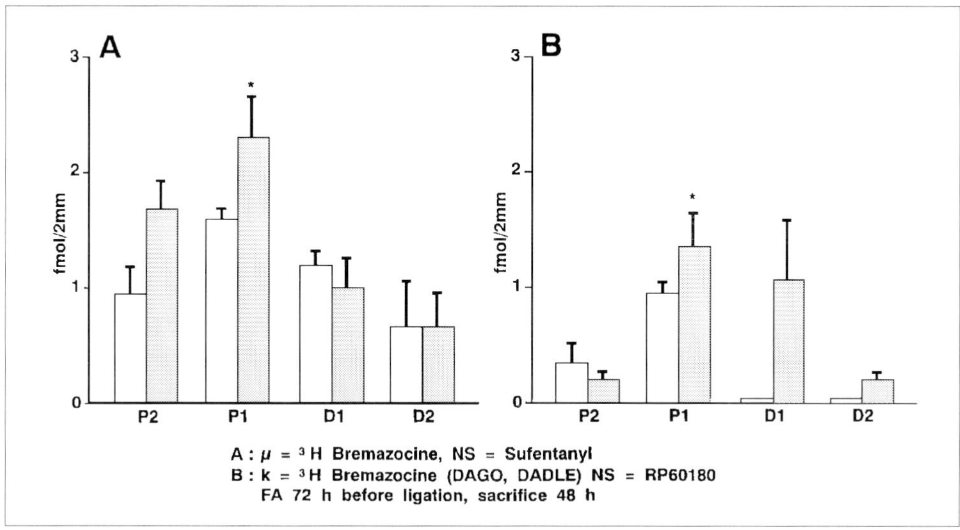

Figure 2. Anterograde and retrograde transport of µ- and κ-receptors in the sciatic nerve. Accumulation of tritiated ligands on both sides of the ligature (P1, D1). (From [7].)
Open bar = normal paw ; black bar : inflamed paw.

is seen in the D1 and D2, possibly because of a lower sensitivity of the κ-binding. If the animals are inflamed, this accumulation close to the ligature is further increased and this is evidenced for the µ- as well as for the κ-receptors. The conclusion from this is that opioid receptors undergo an anterograde transport from the dorsal root ganglion to the periphery and also a retrograde transport from the periphery to the dorsal root ganglion. A further increase is seen in the inflammatory situation and this increase of the opioid receptors at the periphery may explain why these ligands are more active in inflammatory conditions than in normal conditions.

Figure 3 represents a C-afferent fibre which goes to the dorsal horn neuron and makes synapse with an inter-neuron in the dorsal horn. In the peripheral endings enkephalin, dynorphin and opioid receptors are present. Inflammation produces activation of the inter-neuron and then activation of the central pathway. A drug like a κ-opioid may interact with these receptors and thus produces an inhibition of the firing up to the spinal cord. This has been demonstrated by Haley *et al.* [8]. They have recorded single dorsal horn neurons. When formalin is injected at the periphery of the paw, firing is increased in two phases, one which corresponds to the acute activation of the C-fibres due to formalin and the second phase which corresponds to the liberation of mediators at the periphery. If the κ-agonist U-50,488H is injected in the same paw at the very low dose of 100 µg, which is not systemically active here, this produces a total inhibition of the firing at the dorsal horn level. This pharmacological activity of the opioid ligands may be mimicked in some circumstances in more physiological conditions by dynorphin or enkephalins released from the fibres or the immune cells

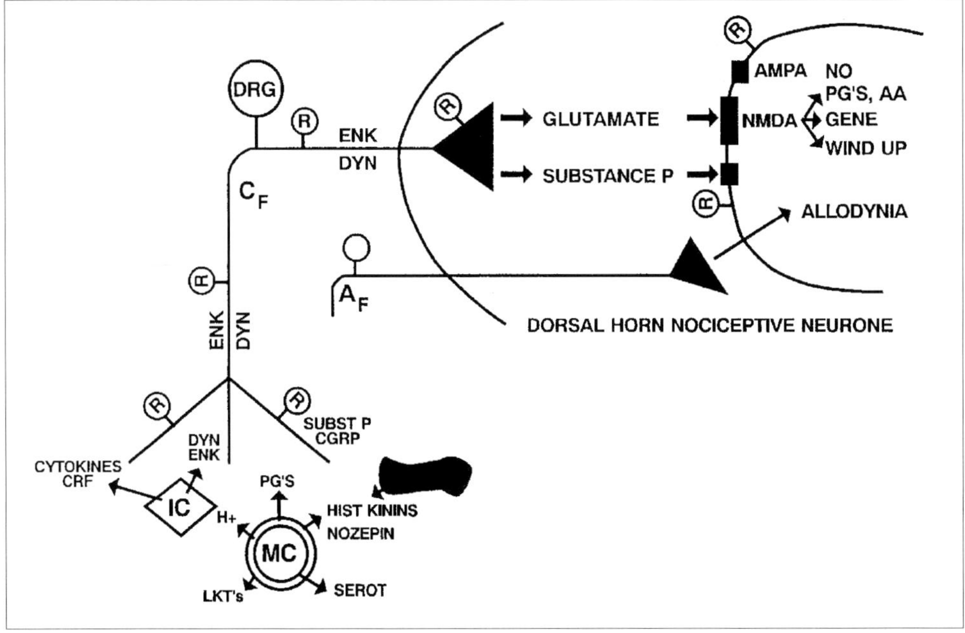

Figure 3. Schematic representation of the primary afferent pathway.
SEROT : serotonin, LKT's : leukotrienes, PG'S : prostaglandins, HIST : histamine, NOZEPIN : norepinephrine, CRF : corticotropin releasing factor, DYN : dynorphin, ENK : enkephalins, IC : immun cell, CGRP : calcitonin gene related peptide, SUBST P : substance P, R : opioid receptor, C_F : C-fibre, DRG : dorsal root ganglia, AMPA : D, L-α-amino-3-hydroxy-5-methyl-4-isoxalone propionic acid, NO : nitric oxyde, AA : arachidonic acid, A_F : A-fibre

present in an inflammatory environment producing some kind of negative feedback loop against the nociceptive response.

What are the evidences for a peripheral site of action of κagonists in visceral pain ? To adress the question, we used two kinds of models in our laboratory, *i.e.* anaesthetized animals to evaluate the nociceptive reflex, and awake animals to assess pain. When animals were anaesthetized, a nociceptive reflex such as hypotension was produced by distension of the gut. A distension of the colon or the duodenum of the rat produces hypotension which can be repeated several times and used for studying efffects of drug [9,10]. We used a distension of 100 mmHg in the duodenum or 75 mmHg in the case of the colon. Hypotension produced by colonic distension was blocked by morphine, the μ-agonist, or U-50,488H, the κ-agonist. When morphine was used at 1 mg/kg i.v., a 100% inhibition of this reflex was obtained, and this could be reversed by a low as well as a high dose of naloxone. In contrast, the κ-selective antagonist nor-BNI did not block the effect of morphine which indicates an effect through the μ-receptors. U-50,488H also blocked the nociceptive response reflex at 100%, but its effect was not blocked by a low dose of naloxone. It was blocked by a universal blocking dose of naloxone, and reversed by the selective antagonist nor-BNI, indicating that κ-receptors are involved.

Where do these effects occur ? To answer the question, we have used different routes of administration (Table I). We administrated morphine and the κ-drug U-50,488H and fedotozine either by i.v. route, by i.c.v. administration directly into the brain or by intrathecal (i.t.) administration in the spinal cord. When morphine was injected into the brain by i.c.v. route, the ED_{50} was found 2 µg per rat, which corresponds to an ED_{50} almost 80 times lower than the one obtained after i.v. administration. In the case of i.t. administration, this ratio was slightly less, the ED_{50} was about ten times lower than the ones by i.v. administration. In other way, this indicates that the main site of action of morphine is supra-spinal. For U-50,488H, the κ-agonist drug, the IC50, after i.c.v. administration was similar to the one determined after i.v. administration, and this is in contrast with what happened with morphine. The ratio between the two ED_{50} is around 1. The same trend occurs after i.t. administration since up to 100 µg which represents more than half the ED_{50} after i.v. route, no activity is found. This indicates that the main site of action of U-50,488H is outside the brain, outside the spinal cord, and this is confirmed by fedotozine which is active after i.v. administration, but does not show activity after i.c.v. or i.t. administration at a dosage which is more than half the ED_{50} after i.v. administration.

Table I. Colonic distension in anaesthetized rats.

Agonist	i.v. (mg/kg)	ED_{50} i.c.v. (µg/rat)	i.t.(µg/rat)	Ratio i.v./i.c.v.
Morphine	0.34 (0.25-0.47)	1.68 (0.84-3.36)	7.73 (3.26-18.31)	81
U-50,488H	0.35 (0.19-0.67)	167 (38-759)	>100	0.83
Fedotozine	2.01 (1.15-3.39)	>300	>300	-

(75 mmHg, 30 sec, 5 min interv., 20 min)

So we were then interested to study the activity of these drugs in a model where pain is measured. We used awake rats instead of anaesthetized rats [11]. We applied to these rats a distension of the rectocolon at a pressure which is not noxious by itself. We applied to these rats a distension of 30mmHg during 10 minutes. In this case there is no pain behaviour. In contrast, if the animals are pre-treated one hour before by an injection of acetic acid in the colon which produces inflammation, the same distension pressure produces pain which can be easily measured by counting abdominal constrictions. The same animals can be challenged 40 minutes later giving the same response. This allows to inject drugs in between the two determinations using the same animals as controls (Table II).

Table II. Distension of the irritated colon in conscious rats.

Agonist	ED_{50} s.c.(mg/kg)	i.c.v.(μg/rat)	Ratio s.c./i.c.v.
Morphine	0.23 (0.09-0.59)	1.70 (0.7-4.3)	47
U-50,488H	0.51 (0.20-1.32)	108 (43.7-270.6)	1.6
Fedotozine	0.67 (0.20-2.23)	>300	<1

(75 mmHg, 30 sec, 5 min interv., 20 min)

μ- and κ-agonists have been injected s.c. Morphine was obviously active after s.c. administration, but the κ- drugs PD-117,302, U-50,488H and fedotozine were as much active. The ED_{50} was in the range of 0.1 to 1 mg/kg. Again this activity was differently mediated in terms of receptors and site of action since morphine again injected i.c.v. was much more active with an ED_{50} which was 50 times lower than the one obtained after s.c. administration while the effect of U-50,488H was almost the same after i.c.v. and s.c. administration. Fedotozine had no activity after i.c.v. administration. Obviously the κ-drugs act on a site which is outside the brain, probably in the peripheral system

Is there any evidence that pain-induced motility and transit anomalies produced by pain can be reversed by peripheral κ-agonists ? Motility or transit anomalies can be induced by injecting acetic acid into the peritoneal cavity of rats and the gastric emptying was determined by using a nutritive meal labelled with 51 chromium [12,13]. After acetic acid administration, the transit was decreased by about 50%. When animals were pretreated with κ-drugs such as U-50,488H, bremazocine or fedotozine, a complete reversion of this inhibition was observed while the μ-agonist, morphine and fentanyl were ineffective or even worsen the transit disturbances (Figure 4). All the κ-ligands we have tested had an activity both on gastric emptying and intestinal transit. This is not shown with fentanyl and morphine, as mentioned before, nor with the prokinetic drug cisapride or some 5HT3 antagonists such as granisetron. In contrast, indomethacin blocks the inflammatory process in the peritoneal cavity.

Fedotozine and U-50,488H were administered by different routes. Using fedotozine up to 300 μg i.c.v. or i.t., we found no reversal in this condition. This again indicates a peripheral site of action of the drug. Recently, Gebhart has provided some elegant experiments showing that these κ-drugs act on the afferent pathways [7]. The firing of pelvic afferent fibres was recorded just before they entered the spinal cord. The afferents were cut at this level and the opioid drugs were injected intra-arterially. Distension of the colon was produced in the presence or in the absence of irritation. When the colon was distended, there was a clear increase of the pelvic afferent firing. When U-50,488H or fedotozine were injected in a cumulative dose, there was an inhibition of this firing

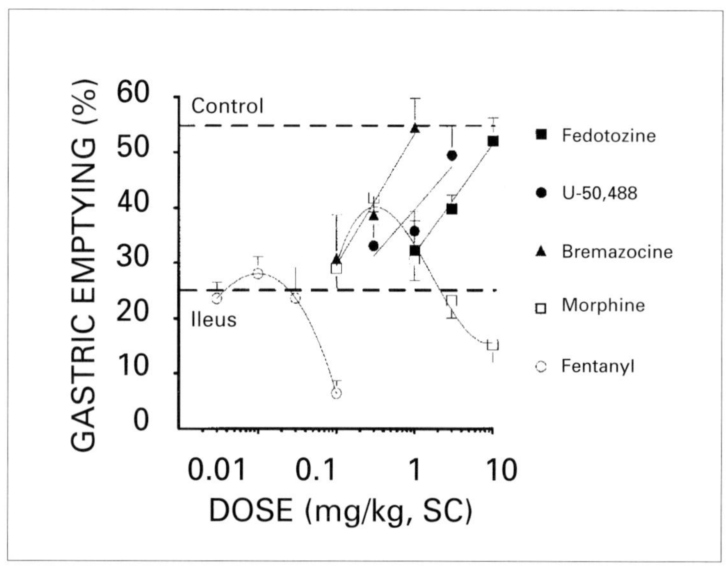

Figure 4. Reversion by κ-ligands of chemically-induced gastric emptying delay.

which was dose-related and this effect can be reversed by a high dose of naloxone, which indicates that this effect of the κ-drugs is opioid receptor-mediated. κ-ligands act at the periphery on the primary afferent fibres.

In conclusion, (a) κ-agonists may exert antinociception through a peripheral mechanism of action, (b) κ–agonists are more active in inflamed *versus* non-inflamed tissues, (c) pharmacological as well as electrophysiological and immunohistochemical data support an effect through opioid receptors located at the distal end of the sensory nerves, (d) κ-agonists can reverse motility and transit anomalies produced by visceral pain while they have no effect on gut functioning in control conditions. These results indicate that peripherally active κ-agonists offer a new approach for treating visceral pain and functional bowel disorders.

References

1. Ferreira SH, Nakamura M. Prostaglandin hyperalgesia II: the peripheral analgesic activity of morphine, enkephalins and opioid antagonists. *Prostaglandins* 1979 ; 18 : 191-200.
2. Joris JL, Dubner R, Hargreaves KM. Opioid analgesia at peripheral sites: a target for opioids released during stress and inflammation. *Anesth Analg* 1987 ; 66 : 1277-81.
3. Stein C, Gramsch C, Herz A. Intrinsic mechanisms of antinociception in inflammation: local opioid receptors and β-endorphin. *J Neurosci* 1990 ; 10 : 1292-8.
4. Stein C, Millan MJ, Shippenberg TS, Peter K, Herz A. Peripheral opioid receptors mediating antinociception in inflammation. Evidence for involvment of mu, delta and kappa receptors. *J Pharmacol Exp Ther* 1989 ; 248 : 1269-75.

5. Hassan AHF, Abletiner A, Stein C, Herz A. Inflammation of the paw enhances axonal transport of opioid receptors in the sciatic nerve and increases their density in the inflamed tissue. *Neurosci* 1993 ; 55 : 185-95.

6. Laduron P. Axonal transport of opiate receptors in capsaicin sensitive neurones. *Brain Res* 1984 ; 294 : 157-60.

7. Sengupta JN, Gebhart GF. Effect of kappa opioid receptors agonists on mechanosensitive pelvic nerve afferent fibers innervating the colon of the rat. *Gastroenterology* 1995 ; 108 : A686.

8. Haley J, Ketchum S, Dickenson A. Peripheral kappa-opioid modulation of the formalin response: an electrophysiological study in the rat. *Eur J Pharmacol* 1990 ; 191 : 437-46.

9. Diop L, Rivière P, Pascaud X, Junien JL. Peripheral kappa-opioid receptors mediate the antinociceptive effect of fedotozine on the duodenal pain reflex in rat. *Eur J Pharmacol* 1994 ; 271 : 65-71.

10. Diop L, Rivière P, Pascaud X, Dassaud M, Junien JL. Role of vagal afferents in the antinociception produced by morphine and U-50,488H in the colonic pain reflex in rats. *Eur J Pharmacol* 1994 ; 257 : 181-7.

11. Langlois A, Diop L, Rivière PJM, Junien JL. Fedotozine inhibits abdominal constrictions induced by colonic distension during colonic hypersensitivity in conscious rats. *Neurogastroenterol Motil* 1994 ; 6 : 140.

12. Rivière P, Pascaud X, Chevalier E, Le Gallou B, Junien JL. Fedotozine reverses ileus by surgery or peritonitis. Action at peripheral kappa opioid receptors. *Gastroenterology* 1993 ; 104 : 724-31.

13. Rivière PJM, Pascaud X, Chevalier E, Junien JL. Fedotozine reversal of peritoneal-irritation-induced ileus in rats ; possible peripheral action on sensory afferents. *J Pharmacol Exp Ther* 1994 ; 270 : 846-50.

Second session

Fedotozine activity on sensitive alterations

Sensitive gastrointestinal disorders. J.P. Galmiche, B. Fraitag.
John Libbey Eurotext, Paris © 1995, pp. 33-41

5

Fedotozine reversion of digestive motility disturbances in ileus. Action on sensory pathways through peripheral kappa receptors

P.J.M. RIVIÈRE, X. PASCAUD, J.L. JUNIEN

Institut de Recherche Jouveinal, Fresnes, France.

Ileus consists in an inhibition of gastrointestinal transit due to a digestive motility impairment. This syndrome may occur after abdominal surgery. Patients with this disorder accumulate gas and secretions, leading to bloating, distension, emesis and visceral pain [1]. Ileus can be experimentally induced in rats by either abdominal surgery or peritoneal irritation [2-5]. In these conditions small intestinal motility [3, 5] as well as gastrointestinal transit are markedly inhibited. Furthermore, motility and transit disturbances are associated with pain as shown by the presence of abdominal contractions. Both models of ileus, abdominal surgery or peritoneal irritation, involve the activation of an extrinsic inhibitory nervous control of gastrointestinal motility [1]. This pathway involves sensory afferents [4], receptors of the corticotropin releasing factor (CRF) in the central nervous system [6, 7] and inhibitory adrenergic efferents [2].

It is well known that both κ- and μ-opioid receptor agonists are able to block pain induced by peritoneal irritation in rodents. However, until recently, no data was available regarding the respective ability of κ- and μ- agonists to reverse motility and transit disturbances associated with abdominal pain in experimental ileus. This paper reviews the effects in ileus of fedotozine, a newly designed peripherally acting κ-opioid agonist which displays high affinity and selectivity for a κ_1- receptor subtype (κ_{1A}) [8].

Material and methods

The techniques used were previously described in details [7, 9, 10]. Briefly, abdominal surgery was performed in anesthetized rats. It consisted in a laparotomy followed by a light caecum palpation (30 s). Peritoneal irritation was induced in conscious rats by intraperitoneal (i.p.) administration of acetic acid (0.6% w/v, 10 ml/kg). Jejunal motility was recorded by electromyography using chronically implanted intraparietal electrodes. Gastric emptying and intestinal transit were evaluated using a liquid nutritive meal (1.5 ml of whole cow milk) labelled with EDTA-^{51}Cr. The meal was administered by gavage 35 min after ileus induction. The animals were sacrificed 15 min later to determine gastric emptying and intestinal transit. Abdominal pain was scored by counting the number of abdominal contractions during the 50 min following ileus induction. Drugs were given by intravenous (i.v.), subcutaneous (s.c.), intracerebroventricular (i.c.v.) or intrathecal (i.t.) route 5 min after ileus induction.

Results

Ileus-induced digestive motility inhibitions

Both abdominal surgery and peritoneal irritation resulted in a marked and long lasting inhibition of small intestinal motility in fasted rats (Figure 1). Fedotozine (3 mg/kg, i.v.) reversed the motility inhibition and restored an almost normal motility pattern in both models. The effects of fedotozine were partly mimicked by U-50,488H, a reference κ-agonist [9]. By contrast, the μ-agonist morphine failed to reverse ileus-induced motor disturbances [9]. Similarly, prokinetic compounds such as cisapride or metoclopramide were also inactive [9].

Ileus-induced gastrointestinal transit inhibitions

In addition to digestive motility disturbances, peritoneal irritation produced an inhibition of about 50% in both gastric emptying (Figure 2) and small intestinal transit [9]. Gastric emptying (Figure 2) as well as small intestinal transit [9] inhibitions were reversed in a dose related manner by fedotozine (ED$_{50}$: 2.4 and 1.8 mg/kg, s.c., for reversion of gastric emptying and small intestinal transit inhibitions, respectively). Fedotozine reversion of ileus was obtained within a dose-range that does not alter basal gastric emptying (Figure 3) or intestinal transit [9] in normal rats. Like fedotozine,

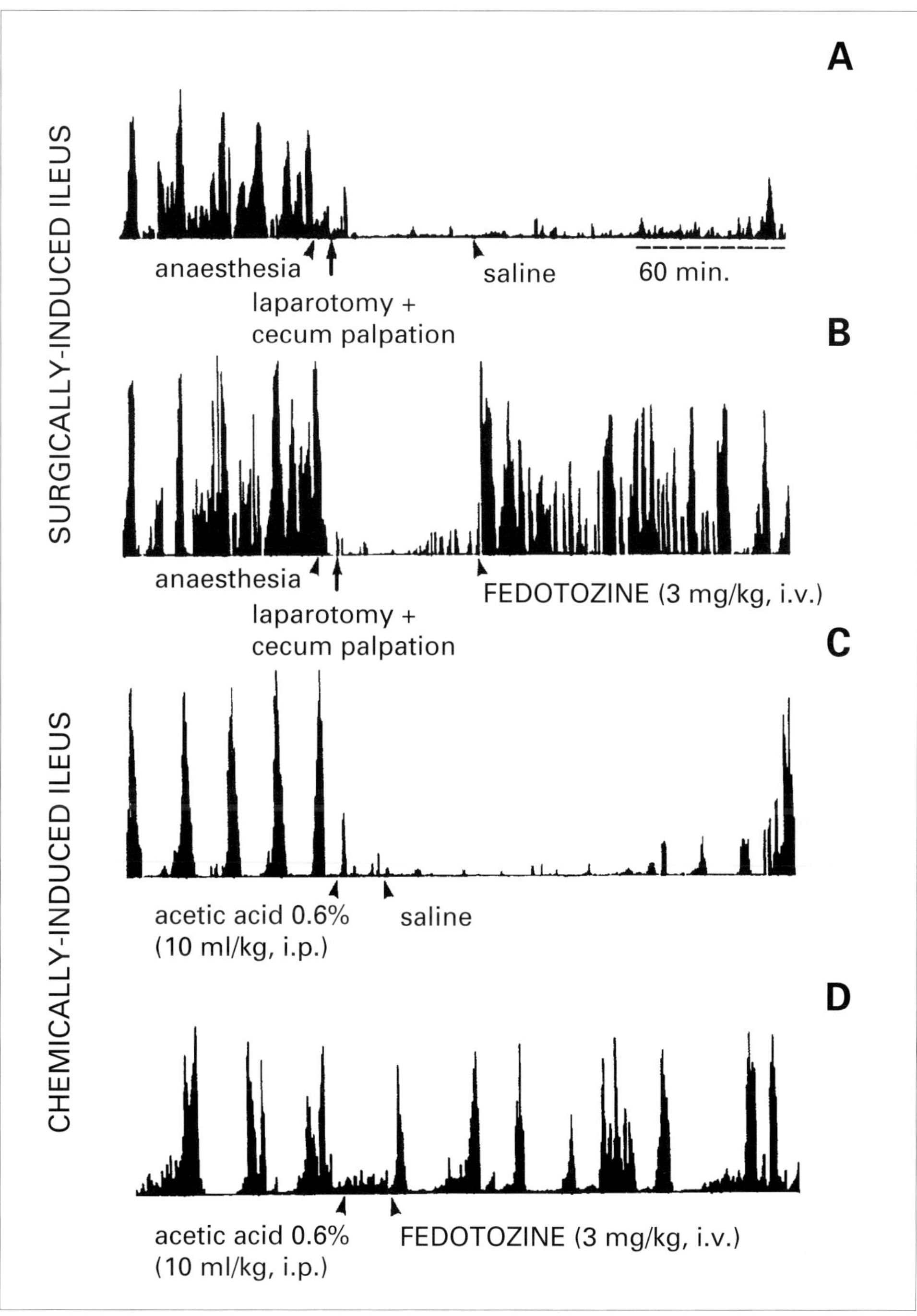

Figure 1. Fedotozine reversion of small intestinal motility (integrated jejunal myoelectrical activity) inhibitions induced by either abdominal surgery (A and B) or peritoneal irritation (C and D). (From [9].)

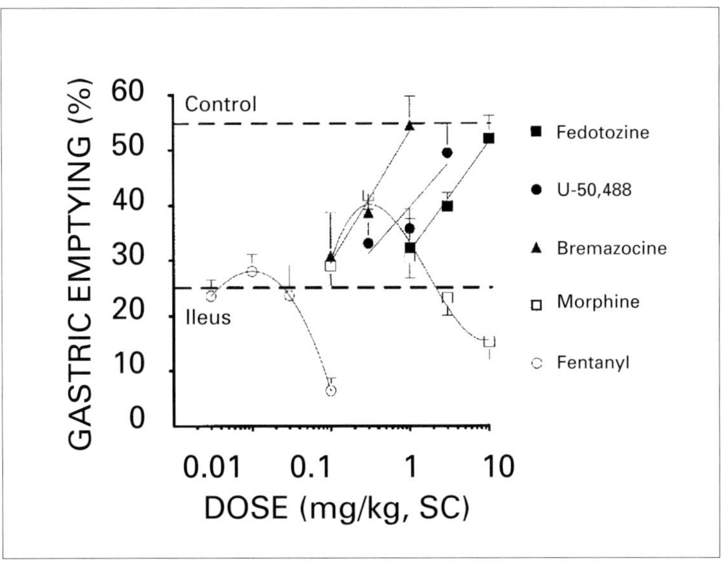

Figure 2. Reversion by fedotozine and reference κ-agonists (U-50,488H, bremazocine), but not by μ-agonists (morphine, fentanyl), of the gastric emptying delay induced by peritoneal irritation. The horizontal dotted lines represent the average gastric emptying in control conditions and after peritoneal irritation induced ileus. (From [9].)

U-50,488H also reversed ileus-induced gastrointestinal transit inhibitions (Figure 2), but failed to alter basal transit (Figure 3). Similar results were obtained with all the reference κ-agonists tested in the model [9, 10]. By contrast, neither fentanyl nor morphine, two μ-agonists, were able to reverse ileus-induced gastrointestinal transit inhibition (Figure 2), which is consistent with their strong antitransit properties in basal conditions (Figure 3). Finally, neither cisapride nor metoclopramide used at doses that have gastrokinetic properties in normal rats were able to reverse ileus [9].

Ileus-induced abdominal pain

Peritoneal irritation induced ileus was also associated with pain that was scored by counting abdominal contractions [10]. This noxious response was inhibited in a dose-related manner by fedotozine within the same dose range used to reverse motility and gastrointestinal transit inhibitions (Figure 4). All the κ-agonists tested in the model also produced a potent antinociceptive activity [10]. Additionally, it was found with κ-agonists that the more potent the compound was to relieve pain, the more potent it was to reverse ileus. A significant and positive correlation was found between the pain relief potency of κ-agonists and their ability to reverse transit disturbances induced by ileus [10]. Finally, μ-agonists were shown to be potent analgesics [10], despite being inactive against motility and transit disturbances (*see* above).

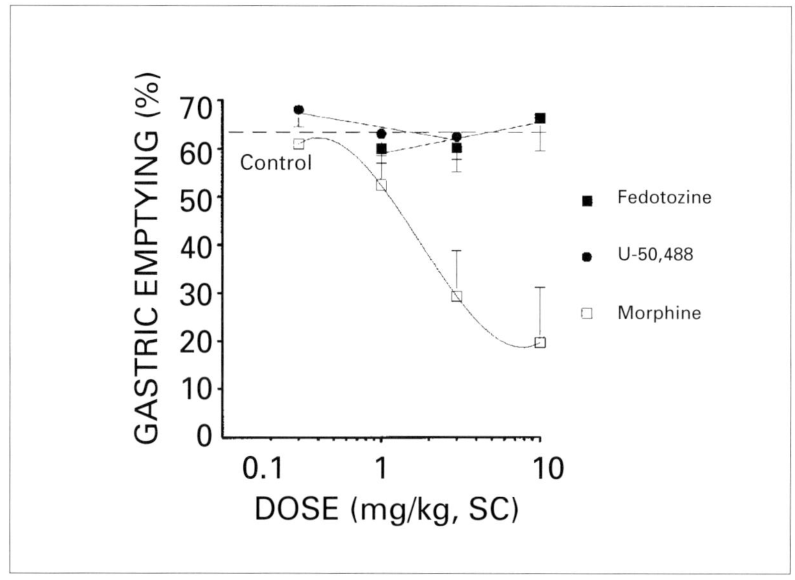

Figure 3. Antitransit activity of morphine compared to the lack of effect of fedotozine and U-50,488H on the basal gastric emptying in normal rats. The horizontal dotted line represents the average gastric emptying in control conditions. (From [9].)

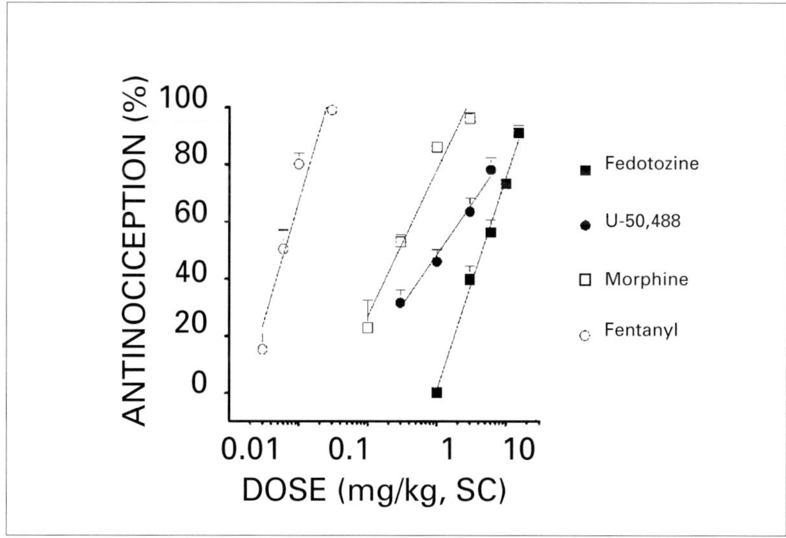

Figure 4. Antinociceptive activity of fedotozine, U-50,488H and reference µ-agonists (morphine, fentanyl) against the noxious reflexes (abdominal contractions) induced by peritoneal irritation. (Adapted from [10].)

Site and mechanism of action of fedotozine in ileus

Peritoneal irritation-induced gastrointestinal transit inhibitions were not reversed by fedotozine given either i.c.v. or i.t. up to 300 µg/rat (Figure 5). This finding suggests that fedotozine responses observed after s.c. administration are due to an action of the compound outside the central nervous system, *i.e.* in the periphery. In agreement with this view, ileus reversion by s.c. fedotozine was prevented by peripheral but not central administration of the opioid antagonist naloxone (Figure 6), suggesting an action at peripherally located opioid receptors. Furthermore, fedotozine response was blocked by the κ-antagonist, nor-binaltorphimine (nor-BNI), indicating an action on κ-opioid receptors (Figure 6). Taken together, the above results support the idea that fedotozine reverse experimental ileus through an action on peripherally located κ-opioid receptors.

Furthermore, central CRF receptors were shown to be involved in peritoneal irritation-induced ileus [7] and exogenous CRF (300 pmol i.c.) was shown to achieve an inhibition of gastric emptying similar in magnitude to that induced by peritoneal irritation [7]. However, neither fedotozine nor U-50,488H were able to reverse CRF induced inhibition of gastric emptying, even at doses that fully block peritoneal irritation-induced ileus (Figure 7). Therefore, in peritoneal irritation-induced ileus, κ-agonists must act before the central activation of CRF receptors, possibly on primary sensory afferent pathways which is consistent with the blockade of pain associated with ileus described here for fedotozine and other reference κ-agonists.

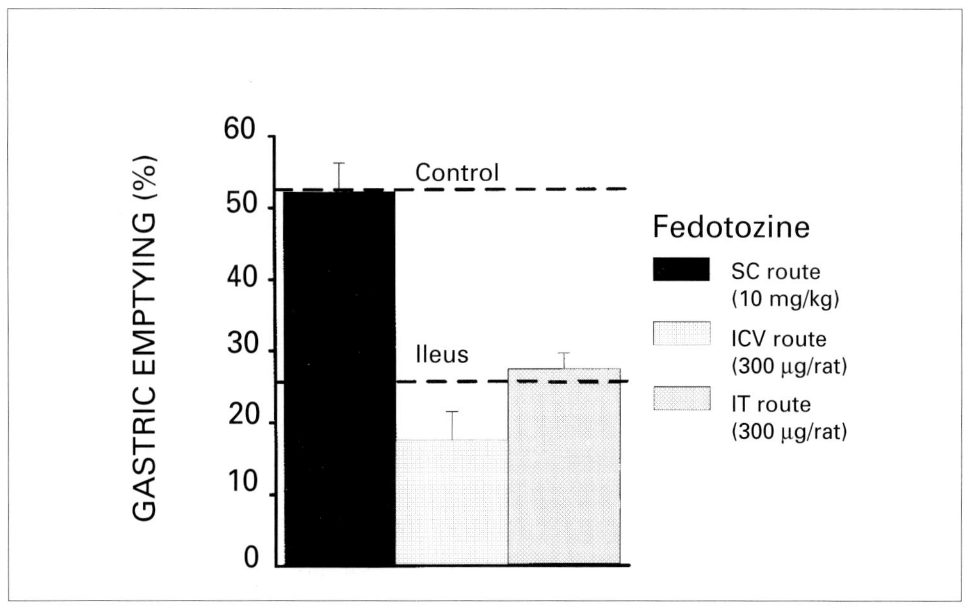

Figure 5. The gastric emptying inhibition induced by peritoneal irritation is reversed by fedotozine when given s.c. but not i.c.v. or i.t. The horizontal dotted lines represent the average gastric emptying in control conditions and after peritoneal irritation-induced ileus. (Adapted from [9].)

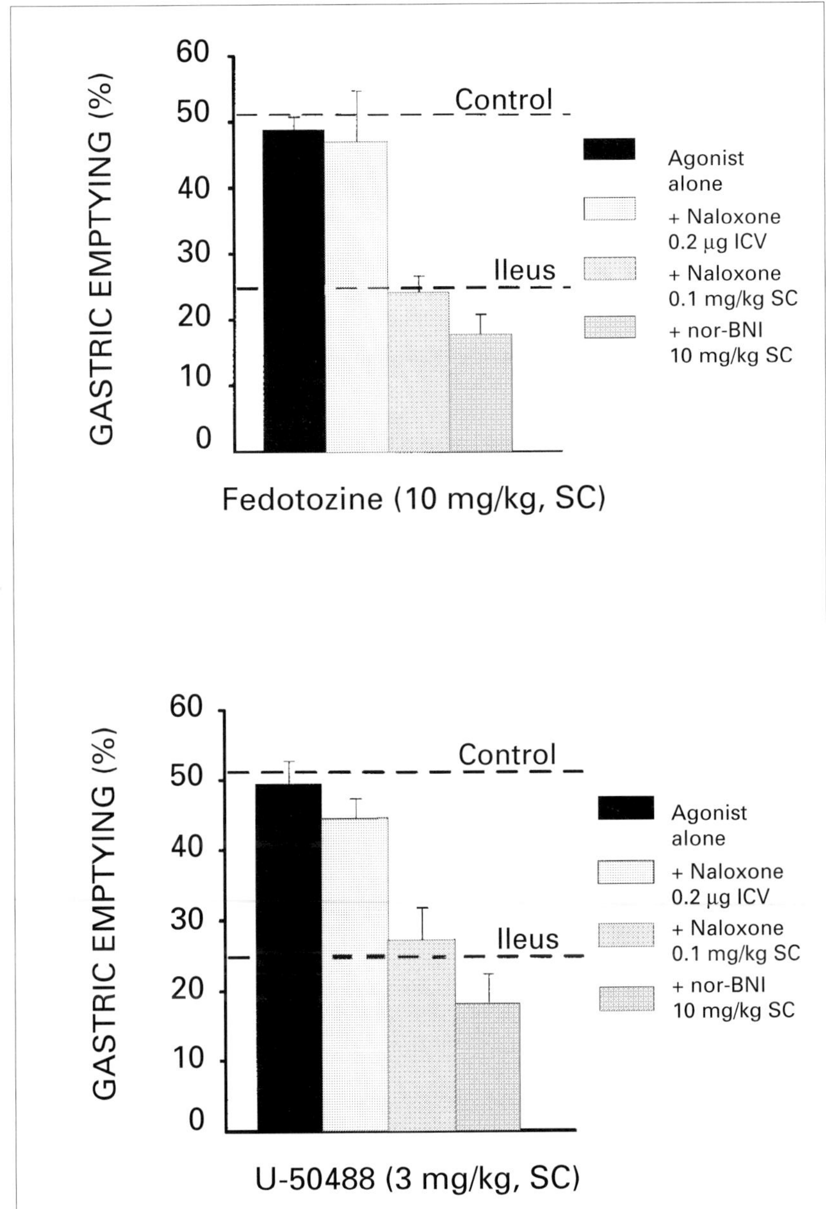

Figure 6. Both fedotozine (top) and U-50,488H (bottom) reversions of the gastric emptying inhibition induced by peritoneal irritation are blocked by the κ-antagonist, nor-binaltorphimine, or by the opioid antagonist naloxone when given s.c. but not i.c.v. The horizontal dotted lines represent the average gastric emptying in control conditions and after peritoneal irritation-induced ileus. (Adapted from [9].)

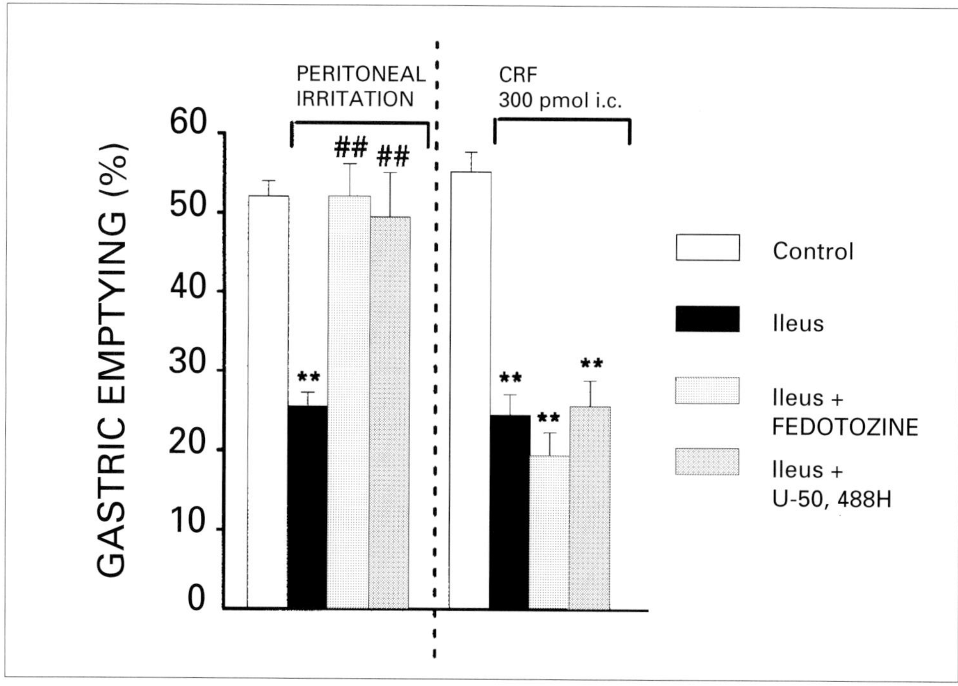

Figure 7. At doses that fully reverse peritoneal irritation-induced inhibition of gastric emptying, neither fedotozine (10 mg/kg, s.c.) nor U-50,488H (3 mg/kg, s.c.) prevented the corticotropin releasing factor-induced inhibition of gastric emptying. Significantly different from **control and ## ileus values, $p \leq 0.01$, Student't test. (Reprinted with kind permission from [7].)

Summary and conclusion

Fedotozine was shown to reverse motility as well as gastrointestinal transit disturbances induced in experimental ileus. This effect is associated with an antinociceptive effect, within the same dose range. Fedotozine responses are observed after peripheral but not central administration, suggesting a peripheral site of action for the compound. Furthermore, fedotozine responses are duplicated by κ-agonists and blocked by a κ-antagonist, suggesting the involvement of κ-receptors. In addition, fedotozine was shown to act on pathways located prior to the activation of central CRF receptors, such as primary sensory afferents. Taken together, the above findings are supporting an action of fedotozine on peripheral κ-receptors that may inhibit nociception transmission at an early stage, *i.e.* on distal ends of visceral primary sensory afferents. Thus, the reversion by fedotozine of ileus-induced motility disturbances seems to be a consequence of an initial action on sensory pathways. Conversely, the lack of activity of prokinetic compounds in this model could be explained by their inability to act on sensory pathways. Furthermore, despite being potent analgesics, μ–agonists failed to reverse motility and transit disturbances, in agreement with their antitransit activity.

In conclusion, it is suggested that κ-agonists such as fedotozine are more appropriated than μ-agonists to treat visceral pain associated with digestive motility and transit disturbances.

References

1. Livingston EH, Passaro EP. Postoperative ileus. *Dig Dis Sci* 1990 ; 35 : 121-32.
2. Dubois A, Weise VK, Kopin IJ. Postoperative ileus in the rat : physiopathology, etiology and treatment. *Ann Surg* 1973 ; 178 : 781-6.
3. Buéno L, Ferré JP, Ruckebush Y. Effect of anaesthesia and surgical procedures on intestinal myoelectrical activity in rats. *Am J Dig Dis* 1978 ; 23 : 690-5.
4. Holzer P, Lippe I Th, Holzer-Petsche U. Inhibition of gastrointestinal transit due to surgical trauma or peritoneal irritation is reduced in capsaicin-treated rats. *Gastroenterology* 1986 ; 91 : 360-3.
5. Sagrada A, Fargeas MJ, Buéno L. Involvement of alpha-1 and alpha-2 adrenoreceptors in postlaparotomy intestinal motor disturbances in the rat. *Gut* 1987 ; 28 : 955-9.
6. Taché Y, Barquist E, Stephens RL, Rivier J. Abdominal surgery and trephination-induced delay in gastric emptying is prevented by intracisternal injection of CRF antagonist in the rat. *J Gastrointest Motil* 1991 ; 3 : 19-25.
7. Rivière PJM, Pascaud X, Chevalier E, Junien JL. Fedotozine reversal of peritoneal irritation-induced ileus in rats; possible peripheral action on sensory afferents. *J Pharm Exp Ther* 1994 ; 270 : 846-50.
8. Lai J, Ma SW, Zhu RH, Rothman RB, Lentes KU, Porreca F. Pharmacological characterization of the cloned kappa opioid receptor as a kappa(1b) subtype. *Neuroreport* 1994 ; 5 : 2161-4.
9. Rivière PJM, Pascaud X, Chevalier E, Le Gallou B, Junien JL. Fedotozine reverses ileus induced by surgery or peritonitis ; action at peripheral kappa opioid receptors. *Gastroenterology* 1993 ; 104 : 724-31.
10. Friese N, Rivière PJM, Chevalier E, Angel-Urban F, Pascaud X, Junien JL. Kappa agonists such as fedotozine inhibit pain and reverse gastrointestinal transit inhibition induced by peritonitis in rats. AGA, New Orleans, May 1994. *Gastroenterology* 1994 ; 106 : A501.

Sensitive gastrointestinal disorders. J.P. Galmiche, B. Fraitag.
John Libbey Eurotext, Paris © 1995, pp. 43-53

6

Fedotozine relieves visceral pain by acting through peripheral kappa receptors. Increased potency during inflammation-induced hyperalgesia in rats

X. PASCAUD, P.J.M. RIVIÈRE, L. DIOP, A. LANGLOIS, J.L. JUNIEN

Institut de Recherche Jouveinal, Fresnes, France.

Fedotozine has been shown *in vitro* to bind to a specific kappa opioid receptor subtype, the κ_{1A} receptor [1], and *in vivo* to reverse motility and gastrointestinal transit disturbances and to block visceral pain in experimental ileus in rats [2-4]. Fedotozine was also shown to reverse antral motility and gastric emptying inhibitions induced by a non painful colonic distension in dogs [5]. All these *in vivo* effects observed after systemic, but not central, administration of fedotozine were reproduced by κ-agonists such as U-50,488H and suppressed by the κ-antagonist, norbinaltorphimine (nor-BNI) or high but not low doses of naloxone. From these results, it was concluded that in these models, fedotozine was acting through peripheral κ-receptors.

The aim of the present study was to extend the concept of visceral pain relief induced by fedotozine in ileus and peritonitis in rats to other models of digestive pain induced by intraluminal distension of the duodenum or the colon in anaesthetized and also in conscious rats.

Material and methods

Animals

Male Sprague-Dawley rats (Iffa Credo, Les Oncins, France) weighing 300-350 g were used. They were housed 3 *per* cage in a regulated environment (20 ± 1 °C ; humidity : 50 ± 5%; light from 8:00 am to 8:00 pm). Food (regular laboratory chow, M25, Extralabo, Piètrement, Provins, France) and water were provided *ad libitum.*

When present, anaesthesia was induced by i.p. injection of pentobarbital (60 mg/kg) and maintained by i.v. infusion of pentobarbital at 12 mg/kg/h. Rats were tracheotomized (polyethylene catheter, id 1.67 mm, od 2.42 mm, Biotrol, France) and a jugular vein and a carotid artery were cannulated (steriflex O.R.X., id 0.5 mm, od 1 mm, Vygon, France) for injection of drugs and monitoring of blood pressure respectively.

For central administration of the drug into the lateral ventricle of the brain (i.c.v.), a polyethylene catheter (PE10 - depth 4 mm) was placed 2 mm lateral and 1 mm posterior to the bregma. Spinal injections were also done using a catheter (PE10) placed in the spinal subarachnoid space at T8 as previously described by Yaksh and Rudy [6]. Location of the end of the catheter was verified at the end of the experiments by injection of Evans blue dye and *post-mortem* examination of the brain and spinal cord.

Pain induction and measurement

Pain was induced by either duodenal (100 mm Hg during 30 sec) or colonic distension (75 mm Hg during 30 sec in anaesthetized rats and 30 mm Hg during 10 min in conscious animals) produced by intraluminal inflation of a 5 cm long latex balloon attached on a polyethylene catheter. In the duodenal pain model, the balloon was inserted through a small opening at the stomach fundus level and kept in position (tip of balloon at 3 cm from the pylorus) by a loose ligature placed around the duodenum (3 cm from the pylorus). In the colonic experiment, the balloon was introduced through the anus and kept in place (tip at 10 cm from the anal verge) by taping the catheter holding the balloon to the base of the tail. Pressure within the balloon was continuously monitored by pressure transducer (Bioblock, Illkrich, France).

In pentobarbital-anaesthetized rats, intraluminal distension induces a reproducible decrease in blood pressure [7]. This stimulus itself was independent of any gut contractile activity that might occur since, in our experimental conditions, a constant pressure distension was applied. None of the drugs tested in this study significantly modified the volume of air required to obtain a constant intraluminal distension pressure indicating that the compliance of the gut wall was not affected and thus did not contribute to a potential antinociceptive effect of the drug tested.

In anaesthetized rats, pain was measured according to Ness and Gebhart [7] by monitoring blood pressure *via* a pressure transducer (P23XL, Gould Electronique, Ballainvilliers, France) and processed by a transducer coupler and amplifier (3B03, Analogue Device, IEF, Issy-les-Moulineaux, France).

In conscious animals, pain was scored by visual counting of abdominal contractions over the 10-min distension period.

Acetic-acid-induced colonic mucosal irritation

Colonic irritation was induced according to the method of McPherson and Pfeiffer [8]. Briefly, 1 ml of 0.6% acetic acid (W/V), or isotonic saline solution in control rats, was introduced at 6 cm from the anal verge into the lumen of the large bowel. At the end of the experiment, the colonic mucosa was examined macroscopically.

Results

Effects of fedotozine on the cardiovascular response to duodenal distension in anaesthetized rats

Under control conditions (n = 48), duodenal distension (100 mm Hg, 30 s) induced a reproducible decrease in blood pressure of 14.04 ± 0.82 mm Hg (Figure 1). Intravenous administration of fedotozine (5 mg/kg i.v.) abolished this response. Its effect was dose-related (Figure 2), the threshold dose being 1 mg/kg and the related ED_{50} was 1.87 (1.1-3.3 mg/kg i.v.). In the same experimental conditions, the ED_{50} values of morphine and U-50,488H were 0.62 and 0.25 mg/kg i.v., respectively (Table I).

Fedotozine administered at a dose of 300 µg/rat (*i.e.* about 0.75 mg/kg) into the lateral ventricle of the brain (i.c.v.) or intrathecally (i.t.) failed to induce any significant inhibition of the blood pressure decrease induced by duodenal distension. U-50,488H (30 to 300 µg/rat i.c.v.) produced a dose-dependent antinociceptive effect but its ED_{50} (149 µg/rat i.c.v.) was close to that found after i.v. administration of the drug. By contrast, morphine (1 to 10 µg/rat i.c.v.) induced a dose-dependent inhibition with an ED_{50} of 2.17 (0.9 - 8.1) µg/rat which corresponds to approximately 1/115 of the i.v. ED_{50}.

Naloxone (30 or 300 µg/kg i.v.) had no effect on the cardiovascular reflex responses induced by painful duodenal distension. Pretreatment with a high (300 µg/kg i.v.) but not low (30 µg/kg i.v.) dose of naloxone blocked the antinociceptive response to fedotozine (5 mg/kg i.v.) and U-50,488H (2 mg/kg i.v.) (Figure 3). By contrast, the lower dose of naloxone was sufficient to abolish the maximal antinociceptive effect of morphine (1 mg/kg i.v.).

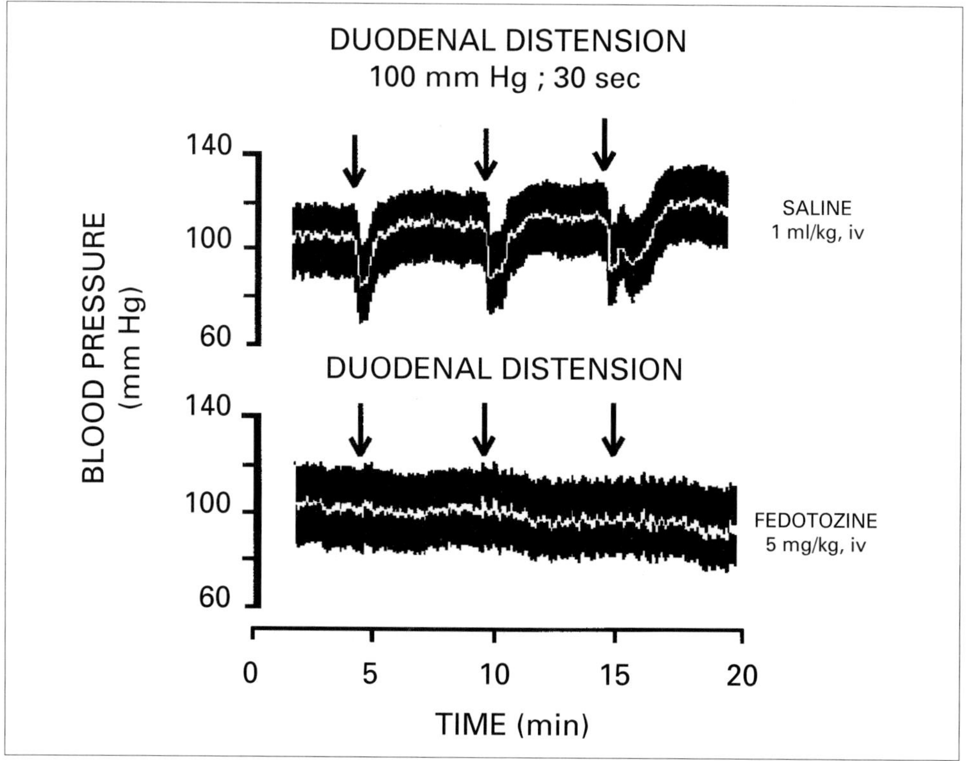

Figure 1. Effect of fedotozine (5mg/kg i.v.) on the reproducible decrease in blood pressure induced by a 100 mmg Hg duodenal distension applied during 30 s.

Table I Comparison of the antinociceptive activities of fedotozine, U-50,488H and morphine given by either s.c. or i.c.v. route on pain induced by duodenal distension in anaesthetized rats.

	ED$_{50}$ values (95% confidence intervals)		
Drugs	**i.v. route (mg / kg)**	**i.c.v. route (μg / rat)**	**Ratio i.v. i.c.v. (*)**
Fedotozine	1.9 (1.1 - 3.3)	>300	
U 50,488H	0.25 (0.1 - 0.6)	2.2	0.6
Morphine	0.6 (0.4 - 1.0)	149 (78 - 283)	115

(*) : To calculate this ratio, i.c.v. doses were expressed as mg/kg

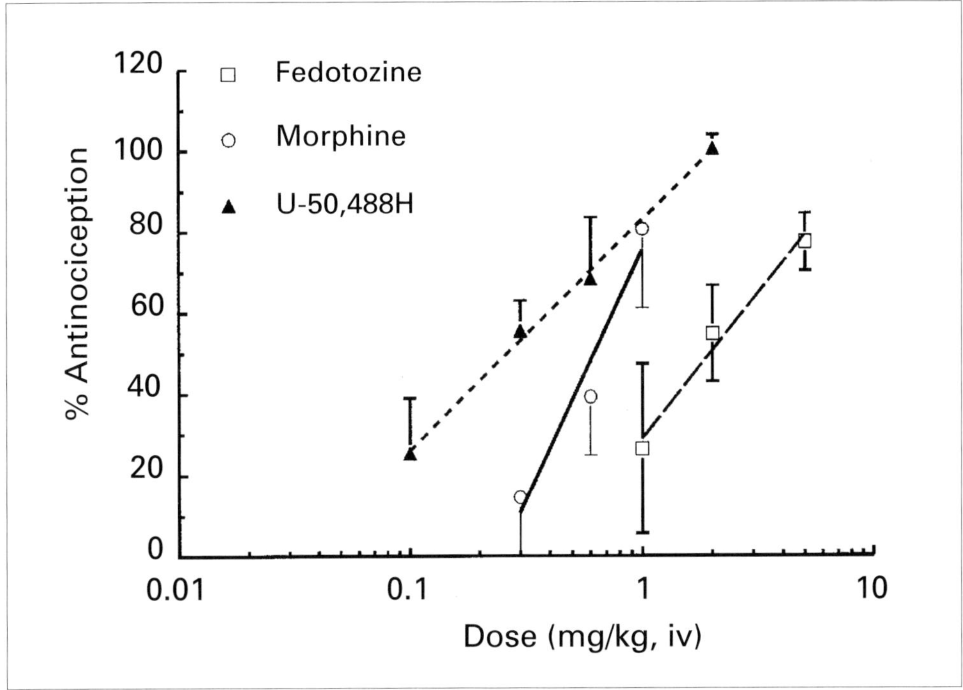

Figure 2. Comparison of the dose-related effects of fedotozine, U50488 and morphine on digestive pain induced by duodenal distension in anaesthetized rat.

The selective κ-antagonist nor-binaltorphimine (10 mg/kg s.c.) did not modify *per se* the cardiovascular reflex response induced by duodenal distension. At this dose, it abolished the antinociceptive effect of fedotozine (5 mg/kg i.v.) and U-50,488H (2 mg/kg i.v.), while it did not significantly modify the response to morphine (1 mg/kg) (Figure 3).

Effects of fedotozine on the cardiovascular response to colonic distension in anaesthetized rats

Preliminary experiments have shown that colonic distension in anaesthetized rats produced a decrease in blood pressure response that correlated well with the increasing intensity of colonic distension, and that the cardiovascular response was enhanced ($p<0.05$) in the acetic acid- *versus* saline- treated rats at each distension pressure applied [9]. A maximal response in both conditions was obtained at 75 mm Hg and this pressure was chosen for the following experiments.

Intravenous injection of fedotozine inhibited the cardiovascular reflex response induced by colonic distension in control and acetic-acid-treated groups in a dose-dependent manner. This activity was greater in the acetic-acid- than in the saline-treated

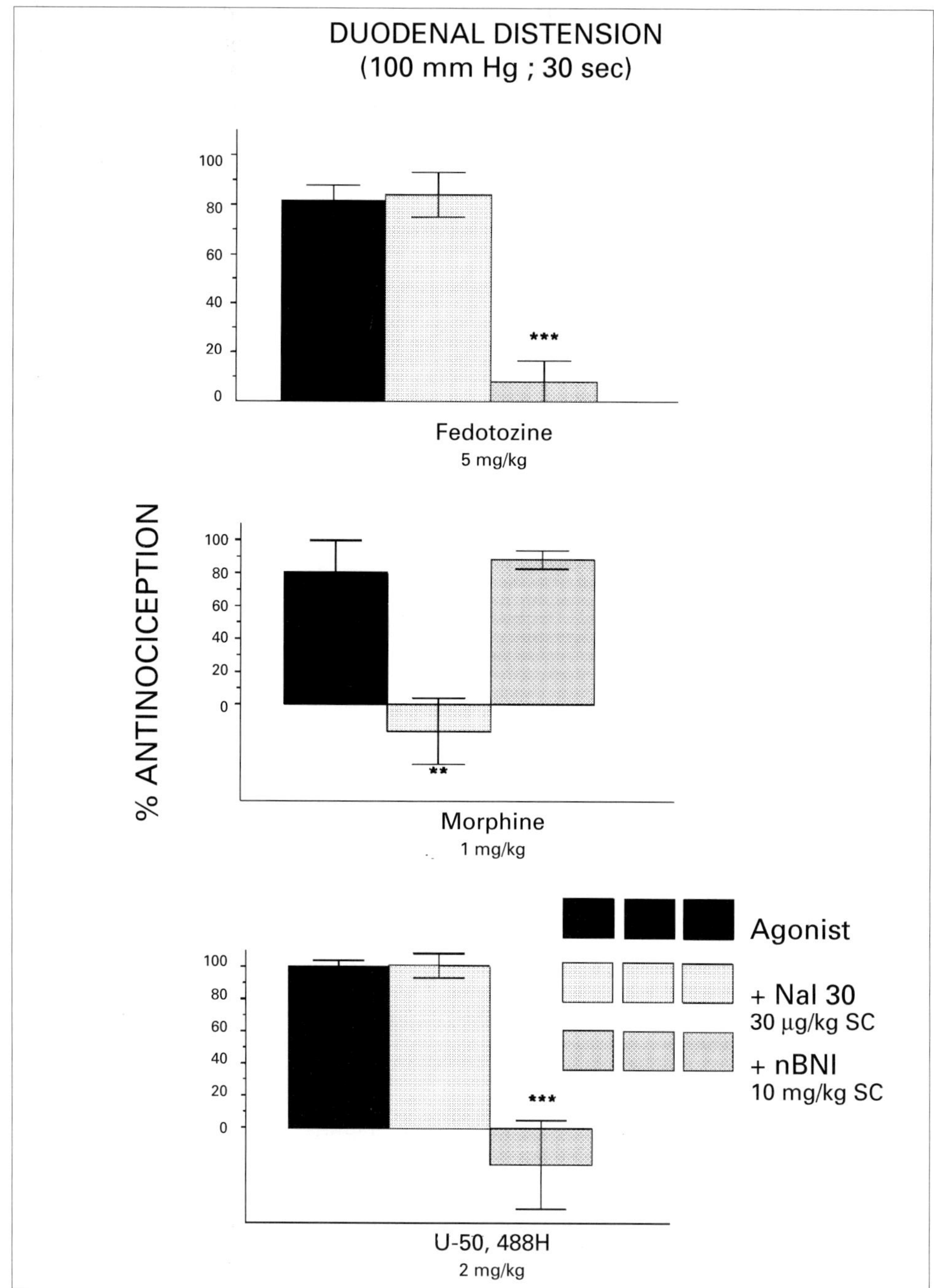

Figure 3. Effect of nalaxone (Nal) and nor-binaltorphimine (nBNI) on fedotozine, U50488 and morphine-induced duodenal pain relief.

group. For instance, at doses of as low as 0.6 or 1 mg/kg i.v., fedotozine was totally inactive in the control group but produced significant antinociceptive activities in the acetic-acid-treated animals (38 and 54 %, respectively, p<0.05), leading to a significantly lower ED_{50} (1.15 *vs* 2.57 mg/kg i.v., p<0.05) (Table II). Similarly, there was a significantly greater antinociceptive response to the selective κ-agonist PD-117,302 in the acetic-acid-treated (ED_{50} : 0.09 mg/kg) than in control rats (ED_{50} : 0.14 mg/kg). By contrast, the antinociceptive effects of morphine remained quite constant in both conditions (0.31 *vs* 0.33 mg/kg i.v. for saline- and acetic-acid-treated groups, respectively).

Table II. Comparison of the antinociceptive activities of fedotozine, U-50,488H and morphine on pain induced by colonic distension in anaesthetized rats with a normal or an irritated colon.

Drugs	ED_{50} mg/kg i.v.		Ratio (*) Irritated/ Normal
	Normal	Irritated	
Fedotozine	2.57	1.15	2.23
PD 117,302	0.14	0.09	1.55
Morphine	0.31	0.33	0.93

(*) : Ratio of the ED_{50} in normal / irritated colon

Effects of fedotozine on the cardiovascular response to colonic distension in conscious rats

In the two previous experiments, digestive pain was measured indirectly in anaesthetized conditions, so the aim of the following experiment was to confirm the antinociceptive activity of fedotozine in conscious animals. Visceral pain was induced by inflating the colonic balloon by 30 mm Hg during 10 min before and 1 h after introducing 1 ml of either saline or 0.6 % acetic acid solution within the colonic lumen, and pain was measured as proposed in the classical writhing test, *i.e.* by counting the number of abdominal contractions induced by the colonic distension.

Such a distension pressure induced a negligible number of abdominal contractions (4.8 ± 1.4 *per* 10 min) in saline-treated rats indicating that it was a pressure threshold beyond which pain can occur (Figure 4). By contrast, the same stimulus induced 23.4 ± 4.1 contractions *per* 10 min (p<0.001) in acetic acid-treated rats indicating that this low pressure became highly painful in those animals.

Fedotozine (0.3 to 3 mg/kg s.c.), given in these conditions of colonic hypersensitivity, dose-dependently decreased the number of abdominal contractions with a potency (ED_{50} : 0.67 mg/kg s.c.) close to that of U-50,488H (ED_{50} : 0.51 mg/kg

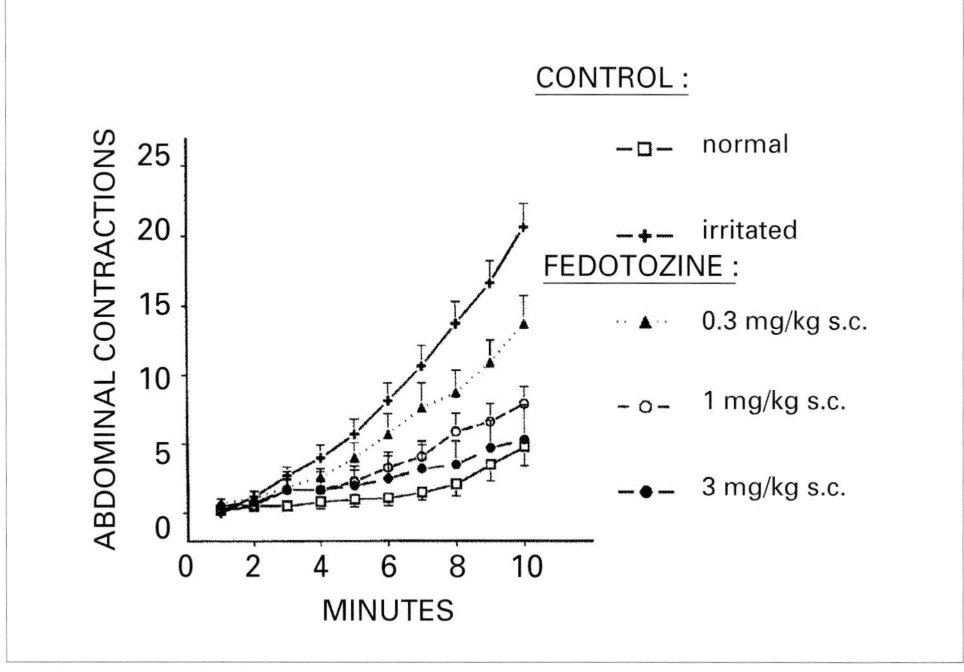

Figure 4. Dose-related effect of fedotozine on pain induced by intraluminal distension applied after colonic irritation induced by acetic acid in conscious rats.

Table III. Comparison of the antinociceptive activities of fedotozine, U-50,488H and morphine administered by s.c. or i.c.v. route on pain induced by colonic distension in conscious rats.

Drugs	ED_{50} (mg/kg s.c.)	Activity (μg/rat i.c.v.)	Ratio s.c./i.c.v. [*]
Fedotozine	0.67	300 = 19%	<1
U 50,488 H	0.51	300 = 58%	<2
Morphine	0.23	ED_{50} = 1.70	47

[*] : To calculate this ratio, i.c.v. doses were expressed as mg/kg

s.c.) and morphine (ED_{50} : 0.23 mg/kg s.c.) (Table III). As already mentioned in the duodenal experiments, fedotozine given in the lateral ventricle of the brain (100 - 300 μg/rat i.c.v.) failed to show any antinociceptive effect. U-50,488H was also poorly effective in these conditions (maximal effect 58% antinociception at 300 μg/rat i.c.v.). By contrast, morphine was 47 times more potent when given centrally (ED_{50} : 1.70 μg/rat i.c.v.) than subcutaneously (ED_{50} : 0.23 mg/kg s.c.).

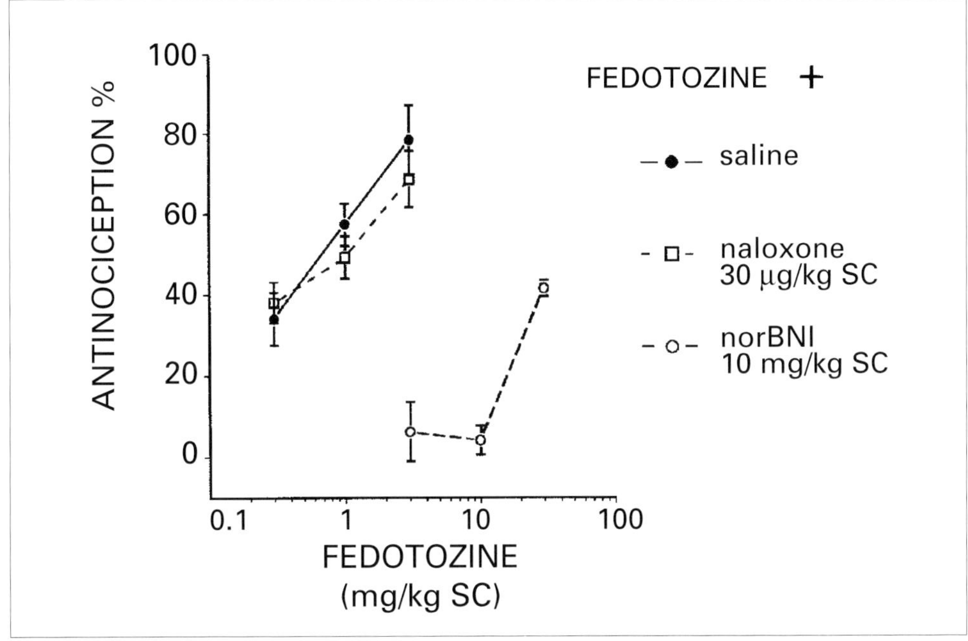

Figure 5. Effect of nalaxone and nor-binaltorphimine in antinociception induced by fedotozine on pain elicited by intraluminal distension of an irritated colon in conscious rat.

Naloxone (30 µg/kg s.c.) used at a dose which abolished the effect of morphine (1 mg/kg s.c.) failed to alter significantly the dose response curve to fedotozine (Figure 5) and did not affect the response to U-50,488H. By contrast, nor-BNI (10 mg/kg s.c.) used at a dose which abolished the effect of U-50,488H and displayed no effect on response to morphine (3 mg/kg), induced a significant right shift of the fedotozine dose-response curve.

Summary and conclusion

In summary, fedotozine used in the same dose range than that used to relieve motility disorders observed in surgical ileus or acetic acid-induced peritonitis in rats [2, 3] was able to inhibit digestive pain induced by intraluminal distension in the upper (duodenum) and lower (colon) gastrointestinal tract. Its effects were reproduced by reference κ-agonists such as U-50,488H or PD-117,302, and also by the µ agonist morphine. However, at variance with morphine that showed a greater potency after central administration, fedotozine was inactive when given into the brain, confirming the strictly peripheral effect of this drug as already described in other models [2, 3, 10, 11].

This antinociceptive activity of fedotozine was blocked by high doses of naloxone, indicating that its effect was driven through opioid receptors, but not by low doses of naloxone which selectively blocked morphine response in the same experiments, indicating that fedotozine effects cannot be related to an action on μ-opioid receptor, consistently with the low affinity of the drug for these receptors. Furthermore, fedotozine antinociceptive effect was blocked by the selective κ-antagonist, nor-binaltorphimine used at doses which abolished the effect of the selective κ-agonist U-50,488H. Taken together, these results support that fedotozine response is due to an action on κ-opioid receptors in agreement with its affinity for this class of opioid receptors.

In conclusion, fedotozine is a powerful digestive pain reliever acting peripherally through κ-receptors. It can be proposed as a new drug in the treatment of functional dyspepsia, irritable bowel syndrome or non-cardiac chest pain in which the common major symptom is known to be altered visceral sensation and pain [12, 13].

References

1. Lai J, Ma SW, Zhu RH, Rothman RB, Lentes KU, Porreca F. Pharmacological characterization of the cloned kappa opioid receptor as a kappa(1b) subtype. *Neuroreport* 1994 ; 5 : 2161-4.
2. Rivière P, Pascaud X, Chevalier E, Le Gallou B, Junien JL. Fedotozine reverses ileus induced by surgery or perionitis: action at peripheral κ-opioid receptors. *Gastroenterology* 1993 ; 104 : 724-31
3. Rivière P, Pascaud X, Chevalier E, Junien JL. Fedotozine reversal of peritoneal-irritation-induced ileus in rats: possible peripheral action on sensory afferents. *J Pharm Exp Ther* 1994 ; 270 : 846-50.
4. Friese N, Rivière PJM, Chevalier E, Angel-Urban F, Pascaud X, Junien JL. Kappa agonists such as fedotozine inhibit pain and reverse gastrointestinal transit inhibition induced by peritonitis in rats. AGA, New Orleans, May 1994. *Gastroenterology* 1994 ; 106 : A501.
5. Gué M, Junien JL, Buéno L. The κ-agonist fedotozine modulates colonic distension-induced inhibition of gastric motility and emptying in dogs. *Gastroenterology* 1994 ; 107 : 1327-34.
6. Yaksh TL, Rudy TA. Chronic catheterization of the spinal subarachnoid space. *Physiol Behav* 1976 ; 17 : 1031-6.
7. Ness TJ, Gebhart GF. Colorectal distension as noxious visceral stimulus: physiologic and pharmacologic characterization of pseudoaffective reflexes in the rat. *Brain Res* 1988 ; 450 : 153-69.
8. Mc Pherson BR, Pfeiffer CJ. Experimental production of diffuse colitis in rats. *Digestion* 1978 ; 17 : 1327-34.
9. Langlois A, Diop L, Rivière PJM, Pascaud X, Junien JL. Effect of fedotozine on cardiovascular pain reflex induced by distension of the irritated colon in the anaesthetized rat. *Eur J Pharmacol* 1994 ; 271 : 245-51.
10. Pascaud X, Honde C, Le Gallou B, Chanoine F, Roman F, Buéno L, Junien JL. Effects of fedotozine on gastrointestinal motility in dogs: mechanism of action and related pharmacokinetics. *J Pharm Pharmacol* 1990 ; 42 : 546-52.
11. Gué M, Junien JL, Pascaud X, Buéno L. Antagonism of stress-induced gastric motor alteration and plasma cortisol release by fedotozine (JO 1996) in dogs. *J Gastrointest Motil* 1990 ; 2 : 258-64.

12. Lémann M, Dederding JP, Flourié B, Franchisseur C, Rambaud JC, Jian R. Abnormal perception of visceral pain in response to gastric distension in chronic idiopathic dyspepsia. The irritable stomach syndrome. *Dig Dis Sci* 1991 ; 36 : 1249-54.
13. Müller-Lissner SA. Functional disorders of the lower gastrointestinal tract. Overview. *Eur J Gastroenterol Hepatol* 1993 ; 5 : 975-8.

Sensitive gastrointestinal disorders. J.P. Galmiche, B. Fraitag.
John Libbey Eurotext, Paris © 1995, pp. 55-63

7

Fedotozine modulates colonic distension-induced inhibition of gastric motility and emptying in dogs

M. GUÉ, L. BUÉNO***

* Institut de Recherche Jouveinal, Fresnes, France.
** Department of Pharmacology, INRA, Toulouse, France.

Background

Motility disorders in different parts of the gastrointestinal tract have been implicated in various functional bowel disorders, such as the irritable bowel syndrome (IBS). Gastric motor disturbances, associated with a delay in gastric emptying, have been described recently in IBS [1], and may result from an inhibitory reflex originating in the colon. Numerous studies have shown that the distension of the colon or the rectum induces a decrease in gastric motility in dogs [2, 3], rats [4], cats [5] and humans [6]. Other studies in human volunteers have shown that painless rectal distension induces an inhibition of postprandial gastric contractions [7] and gastric emptying [8].

Fedotozine is a new compound acting peripherally as an agonist on κ-opioid receptors [9, 10]. Fedotozine as well as κ-agonists restores the gastric migrating motor complex (MMC) inhibited by acoustic stress in dogs by acting on vagal afferents [11] and suppresses the surgical ileus-induced intestinal motor inhibition in rats through peripheral κ-receptors [12].

The aims of this study were to develop a model of non painful prolonged distension of the proximal colon in awake dogs, to determine the effect of distension on gastrointestinal motility in the fasted state, and on gastric emptying of a standard nutritive meal. We further wished to evaluate the influence of fedotozine on the colo-gastric inhibitory reflex on motility and gastric emptying, and to determine its mechanism of action by comparing its effect with U-50,488H (a κ-agonist), and two prokinetics compounds, cisapride and metoclopramide.

Colonic distension during fasted state

Six adult beagle dogs weighing 10-13 kg were used in these experiments. Under halothane (Fluothane ND) anaesthesia, a caecostomy was performed and two strain-gauge transducers implanted using a method previously described [13], one on the stomach, 7 cm from the pylorus and the other on the proximal jejunum, 60 cm from the ligament of Treitz.

Colonic distension and evaluation of pain threshold

Colonic distension was performed using a 10 cm balloon inserted into the colon *via* the caecostomy.

The lowest pressure threshold recorded for visually detectable discomfort and significant ($p \leq 0.05$) increase in heart rate for the six dogs were 44.8 ± 7.2 mm Hg and 50.2 ± 5.9 mm Hg , corresponding to a volume of 90 and 100 ml, respectively (Figure 1). Consequently, in all the experiments, the volume of balloon used was 35 - 40% below the threshold.

Motility studies

In dogs fasted for 20 h, the control antral mechanical activity was characterized by cyclic phases of gastric contractions occurring at 113.4 ± 18.6 min intervals. Colonic distension (60 ml) delayed by 141 % the occurrence of the next gastric MMC, while the jejunal MMC continued at a normal frequency (Figure 2). Compliance curves indicated that, for a volume of 60 ml, colonic pressure was 33.0 ± 5.4 mm Hg (Figure 1). The time interval between the first and second gastric MMC after colonic distension (CD) was not significantly different ($p > 0.05$) from the control interval. No difference in gastric response was observed between naive and previously tested dogs.

Effect of fedotozine and U50 488

When injected at doses of 25 and 50 µg/kg i.v. in fasted dogs, fedotozine did not affect significantly ($p > 0.05$) the duration of the gastric MMC cycle. Injected 10 min

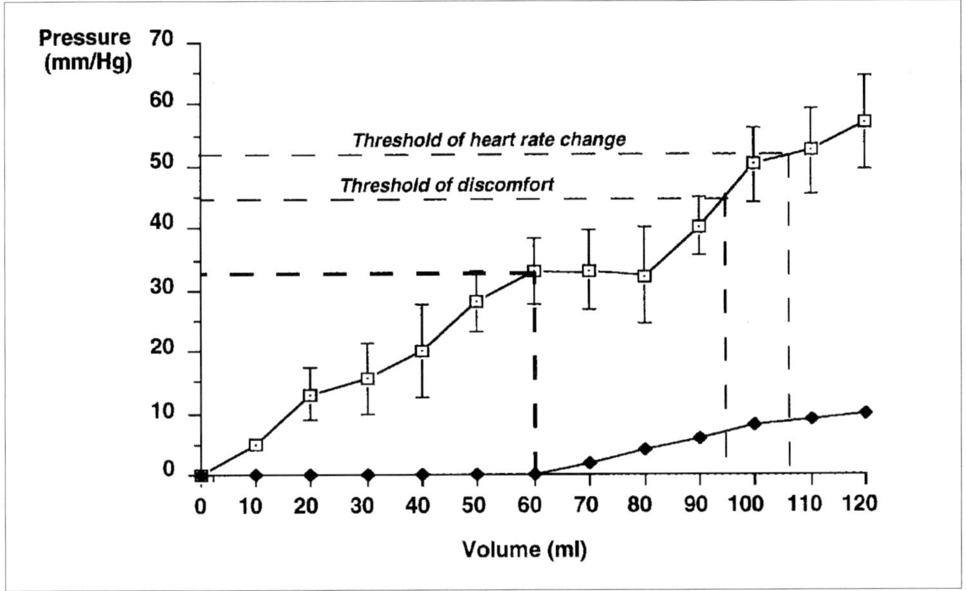

Figure 1. Changes in pressure *vs* volume of balloon on the bench (♦) or inserted into the proximal colon of dogs ([•]). Results are means ± SD; n=12. Dotted lines indicate the lowest volumes at which heart rate changes and discomfort were observed. Note that for a volume of 60 ml, the resistance of the balloon is negligible and that the intraballoon pressure is equivalent to the intracolonic pressure.

before CD, fedotozine (25 and 50 µg/kg i.v.) abolished the CD-induced lengthening of the gastric MMC cycle (Table I and Figure 3) However, at a lower dose (10 µg/kg), fedotozine did not reduce the CD-induced gastric motor changes (Table I). Similarly, U-50,488H also suppressed (p<0.05) the inhibition of gastric MMC induced by CD, at doses of 25 and 50 µg/kg i.v. (Table I and Figure 3), but not for lower dosage (Table I).

Effect of cisapride and metoclopramide

Cisapride and metoclopramide injected i.v. at 10 and 50 µg/kg had no effect *per se* on gastrointestinal motility ; in addition they were inactive on the lengthening of gastric MMC induced by CD (Table I).

Antagonism of fedotozine by nor-binaltorphimine

Injected at a dose of 1 mg/kg i.v., nor-binaltorphimine (nor-BNI) had no effect on gastrointestinal motility and on colonic distension-induced gastric motor inhibition (Table II). However, administered 10 min before fedotozine (50 µg/kg i.v.), nor-BNI abolished the inhibitory action of fedotozine on CD-induced inhibition of gastric MMC (Figure 4).

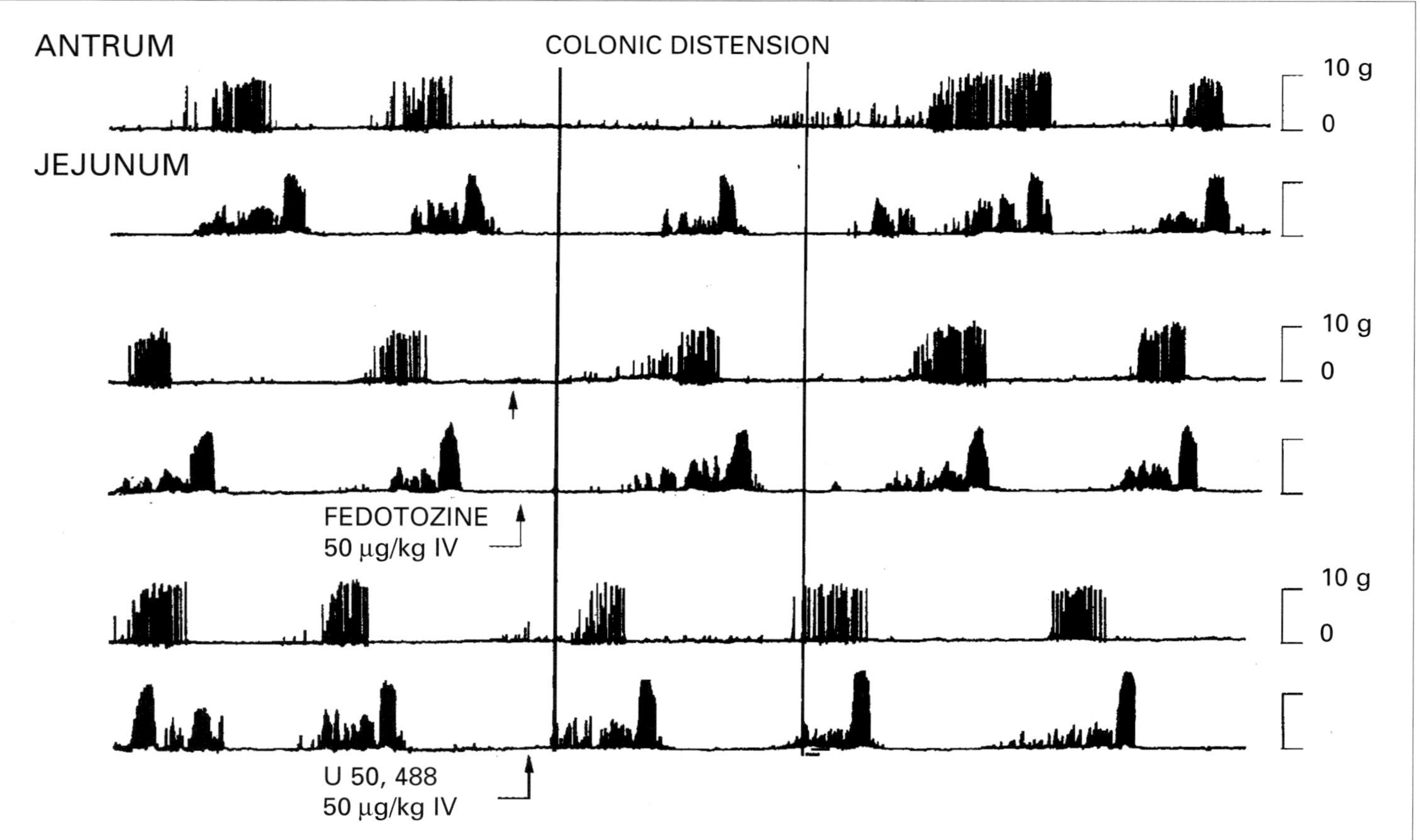

Figure 2. Blockade of colonic distension-induced inhibition of gastric MMC by fedotozine and U 560 488 in fasted dogs. Note that colonic distension selectively delayed the occurrence of the gastric but not the jejunal MMC.

Table I. Effects of fedotozine, U-50,488H, cisapride and metoclopramide on colonic distension-induced inhibition of gastric migrating motor complex in fasted dogs (mean ± SD, n=12 essays).

Drugs (μg/kg IV)	Gastric MMC cycle (min)	
	Basal	**Colonic distension**
Saline (0.5 ml/kg IV)	96.9 = 13.7	233.9 ± 24.3 [*]
Fedotozine		
10	111.5 ± 20.2	229.4 ± 29.5 [*]
25	106.4 ± 20.8	124.9 ± 15.3
50	108.1 ± 20.9	103.9 ± 9.9
U-50,488H		
10	105.3 ± 15.7	215.1 ± 28.4 [*]
25	97.0 ± 10.6	132.8 ± 35.4
50	110.3 ± 21.6	124.9 ± 22.3
Cisapride		
10	112.6 ± 31.4	228.6 ± 21.4 [*]
50	122.3 ± 18.9	243.5 ± 35.8 [*]
Metoclopramide		
10	116.4 ± 19.9	231.4 ± 16.9 [*]
50	106.6 ± 26.3	210.6 ± 38.7 [*]

[*] : significantly (p≥0.05) different from corresponding basal values

Table II. Effect of nor-binaltorphimine (1 mg/kg i.v.) on disinhibition by fedotozine of colonic distension-induced gastric motor inhibition (mean ± SE ; n = 12).

Drugs	Gastric MMC cycle (min)	
	Basal	**Colonic distension**
Control		
Saline (0.5 ml/kg IV)	96.9 ± 13.7	233.9 ± 24.3 [*]
Fedotozine (50 μg/kg IV)	108.1 ± 20.9	103.9 ± 9.9
After nor-BNI		
Saline (0.5 ml/kg IV)	112.3 ± 23.4	239.7 ± 31.5 [*]
Fedotozine (50 μg/kg IV)	91.3 ± 11.7	225.8 ± 33.8 [*]

[*] : significantly (p≤0.05) different from "basal" corresponding values

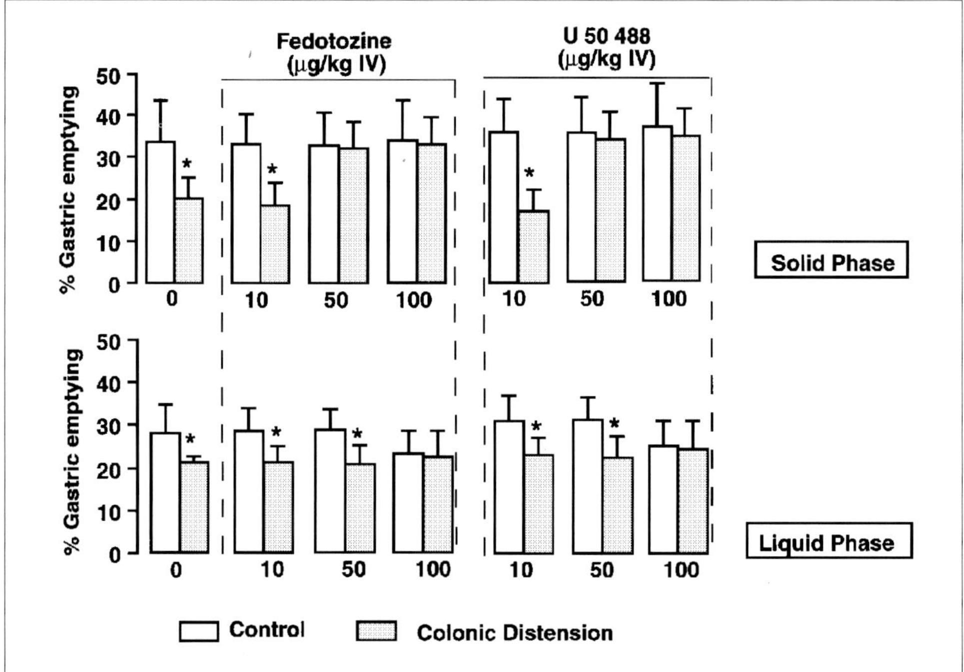

Figure 3. Influence of fedotozine and U 50488 on colonic distension-induced delay in gastric emptying of solids and liquids of a standard meal in dogs.
* : significantly (p < 0.05) different from corresponding basal value by Wilcoxon matched-pair signed-rank test. Results are means ± SD ; n = 12.

Colonic distension on gastric emptying

Four male adult beagle dogs weighing 10-12 kg were used for these experiments; under halothane anaesthesia, a Thomas cannula was placed on the greater curvature of the gastric body at about 10 cm from the pylorus, it was exteriorized on the left abdominal wall 5 cm from the last rib and 10 cm from the midline. A caecostomy was also performed and the animals were allowed to recover for two weeks before tests. The rate of gastric emptying of liquids and solids was calculated following a previously described method [14].

Colonic distension

Under control conditions, the gastric emptying of solids measured 1 hour after feeding was 33.6 ± 9.9 % (mean ± SD, n = 12) of the initial weight of the solid phase and the volume of liquid emptied was 25.8 ± 6.1 % of the initial volume.

CD applied immediately after meal ingestion significantly (p<0.05) inhibited by 40.2 % and 24.8 %, respectively, the gastric emptying of solids and liquids (Figure 3).

Effect of fedotozine and U-50,488H on gastric emptying

When given at doses of 10 to 100 µg/kg i.v., fedotozine did not affect the rate of gastric emptying of solids and liquids. However, pretreatment with fedotozine (50 and 100 µg/kg i.v.) abolished the CD-induced reduction of gastric emptying of solids ; but only the highest dose reduced the inhibitory effect of CD on gastric emptying of liquids (Figure 3). Similarly, U-50,488H (10, 50 and 100 µg/kg i.v.) did not affect the gastric emptying of solids in control conditions ; however, at a dose of 100 µg/kg i.v., U-50,488H reduced the gastric emptying of liquids significantly (p≤0.05). Given 10 min before CD, U-50,488H (50 and 100 µg/kg i.v.) restored the gastric emptying of solids to normal values, but had no effect on the CD-induced delay in gastric emptying of liquids (Figure 3).

Antagonism by nor-binaltorphimine

Nor-BNI (1 mg/kg i.v.) had no effect on gastric emptying and on the CD-induced delay on gastric emptying (Figure 4). However, injected 10 min before fedotozine (50 µg/kg i.v.), nor-BNI restored the delay of gastric emptying induced by CD (Figure 4).

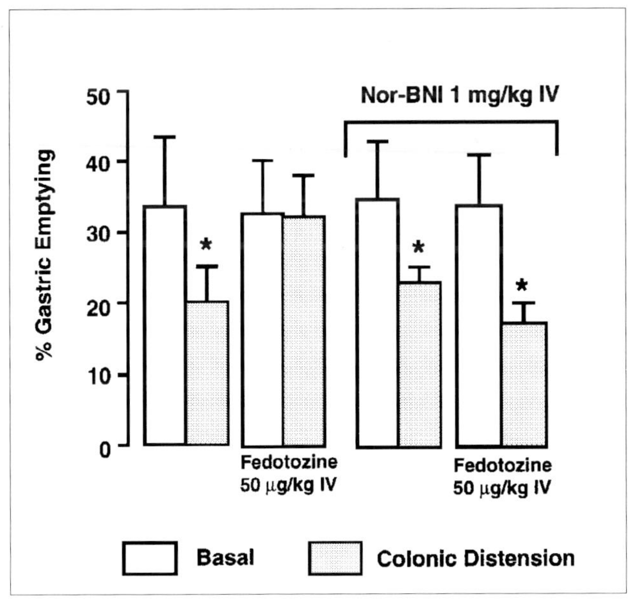

Figure 4. Effect of nor-binaltorphimine on the suppressive effect of fedotozine on colonic distension-induced delay in gastric emptying of solids in dogs.
* : significantly (p< 0.05) different from corresponding basal values.

Discussion

CD below a painful sensation threshold is enough to disrupt the gastric MMC cycle without change in the cyclic occurrence of intestinal MMC. It has been recently found that gastric motility and gastric emptying are delayed in irritable bowel syndrome (IBS) patients [1] and that 50-80% of IBS patients have symptoms suggestive of disturbed gastric emptying [15, 16]. Consequently, this light CD-induced inhibition of gastric motility may be a useful model of the colo-gastric reflex which may contribute to pathophysiological problems in IBS patients. Our method seems to be relevant to study physiopathology of IBS, since the most common symptom described by these patients is a colonic pain, few hours after a meal, associated with the entry of digested food into the colon as indicated by breath hydrogen concentration [17].

Our results show that U-50,488H, a selective κ-receptor agonist, and fedotozine suppress the colo-gastric inhibitory reflex induced by CD, suggesting that fedotozine acts through κ-receptors, an hypothesis confirmed by the antagonism of the suppressive effect of fedotozine by nor-BNI, a selective κ-receptor antagonist [18].

Compounds such as metoclopramide or cisapride, which have prokinetic properties under basal conditions [19, 20], failed to restore normal gastric motility during colonic distension.

In the present study, we also show that a painless CD delays gastric emptying of both solid and liquid phases of a standard meal in dogs ; this result is in agreement with a delayed gastric emptying observed in humans during painless rectal distension [8]. As for the gastric MMC inhibition in the fasted state, the blocking effect of fedotozine on CD-induced delay in gastric emptying is abolished by pretreatment with the κ-receptor antagonist nor-BNI, suggesting that, here again, fedotozine acts through κ-receptors to block the gastric response to CD during the postprandial state. Since recently Van Wijk *et al.*, [1] have shown that IBS patients present a delay in gastric emptying, it could be speculated that fedotozine or U-50,488H will be able to relieve related symptoms presented by IBS patients.

In conclusion, the present work demonstrates that a light colonic distension below painful sensation is enough to suppress gastric MMC in fasted state and to delay gastric emptying and that fedotozine and U-50,488H act through κ-receptors to restore a normal gastric motility and emptying.

References

1. van Wijk HJ, Smout AJPM, Akkermans LMA, Roelofs JMM, ten Thije OJ. Gastric emptying and dyspeptic symptoms in the irritable bowel syndrome. *Scand J Gastroenterol* 1992 ; 27 : 99-102.
2. Pearcy JF, Van Liere EJ. Studies on the visceral nervous system. Reflexes from the colon. *Am J Physiol* 1926 ; 78 : 57-64.
3. Youmans WM, Meak WJ. Reflex and humoral gastro-intestinal inhibition in unanaesthetized dogs during rectal stimulation. *Am J Physiol* 1937 ; 120 : 750-5.
4. Bojö L, Cassuto J. Gastric reflex relaxation by colonic distension. *J Auton Nerv Syst* 1992 ; 38 : 57-64.
5. Jansson G. Vago-vagal reflex relaxation of the stomach in the cat. *Acta Physiol Scand* 1969 ; 75 : 245-52.
6. Zighelboim J, Talley NJ, Camilleri M, Phillips SF. Identification of a recto-gastric response in health using the barostat. *Gastroenterology* 1993 ; A606.
7. Kellow JE, Gill RC, Wingate DL. Modulation of human upper gastrointestinal motility by rectal distension. *Gut* 1987 ; 28 : 864-8.
8. Youle M, Read NW. Effect of painless rectal distension on gastrointestinal transit of solid meal. *Dig Dis Sci* 1984 ; 29 : 902-6.
9. Pascaud X, Honde C, Le Gallou B, Chanoine F, Roman F, Buéno L, Junien JL. Effects of fedotozine on gastrointestinal motility in dogs : mechanism of action and related pharmacokinetics. *J Pharm Pharmacol* 1990 ; 42 : 546-52.
10. Karaus M, Kittelman R, Lubke HJ, Erckenbrecht JF. Selective stimulation of phase 3 activity by fedotozine (JO 1196) in men. *Gastroenterology* 1990 ; 98 : A364.
11. Gué M, Junien JL, Pascaud X, Buéno L. Antagonism of stress-induced gastric motor alteration and plasma cortisol release by fedotozine (JO 1196) in dogs. *J Gastrointest Motility* 1990 ; 2 : 258-64.
12. Rivière PJM, Pascaud X, Chevalier E, Le Gallou B, Junien JL. Fedotozine reverses ileus induced by surgery or peritonitis : action at peripheral κ-opioid receptors. *Gastroenterology* 1993 ; 104 : 724-31.
13. Pascaud X, Genton MJ, Bass P. A miniature transducer for recording intestinal motility in unrestrained chronic rats. *Am J Physiol* 1978 ; 235 : E529-E532.
14. Gué M, Fioramonti J, Buéno L. A simple double radiolabelled technique to evaluate gastric emptying of canned food meal in dogs : application to pharmacological tests. *Gastroenterol Clin Biol* 1988 ; 12 : 425-30.
15. Svendlund J, Sjödin I, Dotevall G, Gillberg R. Upper gastrointestinal and mental symptoms in the irritable bowel syndrome. *Scand J Gastroenterol* 1985 ; 20 : 595-601.
16. Whorwell PJ, Mc Callum M, Reed FH, Roberts CT. Non-color features of irritable bowel syndrome. *Gut* 1986 ; 27 : 37-40.
17. Cann PA, Read NW. A disease of the whole gut ? In : Read NW, ed. *Irritable bowel syndrome*. London : Grune and Stratton, 1985 : 53-63.
18. Portoghese PS, Lipkowski AW, Takemori AE. Binaltorphimine and nor-binaltorphimine, potent and selective κ-opioid receptors antagonists. *Life Sci* 1987 ; 40 : 1287-92.
19. Shuurkes JAJ, Akkermans LMA, Van Nueten JM. Stimulating effects of cisapride on antroduodenal motility in the conscious dog. In : Roman C, ed. *Gastrointestinal motility*. Lancaster MTP Press, 1984 : 95-102.
20. Pinder RM, Brogden RN, Sawyer PR, Speight TM, Avery GS. Metoclopramide : a review of its pharmacological properties and clinical use. *Drugs* 1976 ; 12 : 81-131.

Sensitive gastrointestinal disorders. J.P. Galmiche, B. Fraitag.
John Libbey Eurotext, Paris © 1995, pp. 65-71

8

Effects of fedotozine on mechanosensitive pelvic nerve afferent fibres in the rat

G.F. GEBHART, J.N. SENGUPTA

Department of Pharmacology, University of Iowa, USA.

It has been suggested that the principal site of action of fedotozine is peripheral. The objective of the present study was to directly examine the effects of fedotozine on pelvic nerve afferent fibre responses to noxious colorectal distension in the rat. The results of experiments summarized below clearly document that agonists with actions at the κ-opioid receptor, but not morphine (the μ-opioid receptor-preferring agonist), dose-dependently attenuate responses of pelvic nerve afferent fibres to colorectal distension.

Experiments were performed in deeply anaesthetized rats in which the first sacral dorsal root (S1) was decentralized. Accordingly, any effects of drugs were restricted to a peripheral site of action (*e.g.*, the colon, the afferent fibre terminal or the afferent fibre). Afferent fibres that innervate the colon were located in the decentralized S1 dorsal root by electrical stimulation of the pelvic nerve. The experimental arrangement is illustrated in Figure 1. A 7 cm long latex balloon inserted into the colon *via* the anus was used to distend the colon with air at constant pressure. Distending pressures ranged between 5 and 100 mmHg, 30 sec duration given every 4 min. Drug effects were tested against noxious colorectal distension (80 mmHg). Drugs were given by close intra-arterial injection and drug dosage (reported as the salt) was cumulative in an experiment. The drugs that were studied were morphine (purchased from Mallinckrodt, Paris, KY, USA), fedotozine and U-50,488H (provided by Institut de Recherche Jouveinal). In addition to studying drug effects on pelvic nerve afferent fibres from the normal, uninflammed colon, in some experiments drug effects were studied 30 or 60 min after intracolonic instillation of 2.5% acetic acid (2 ml).

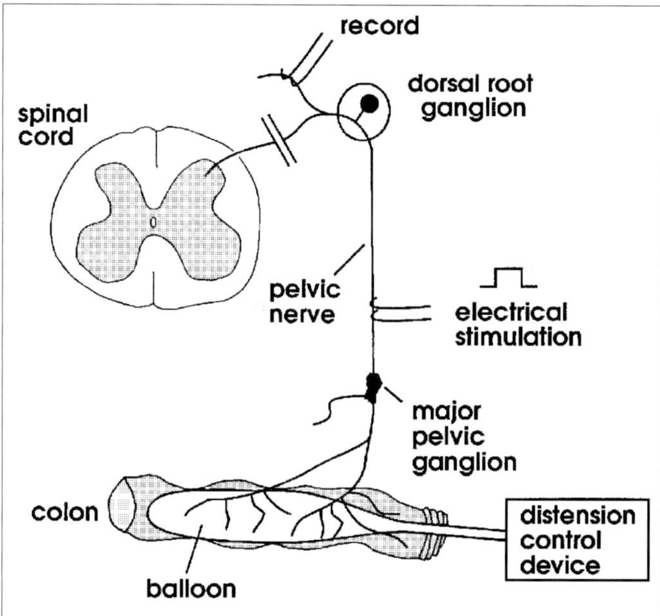

Figure 1. Diagrammatic representation of the stimulation and recording arrangement. The effects of drugs were studied on afferent fibres in the decentralized S1 dorsal root that responded to electrical stimulation of the pelvic nerve (central to the major pelvic ganglion) and to balloon distension of the colon.

After teasing a fibre from the S1 dorsal root and establishing that it responded to electrical stimulation of the pelvic nerve (the search stimulus) and to colonic distension, the threshold for response to colonic distension was determined. In earlier work [1], we determined that there exists both low threshold and high threshold pelvic nerve afferent fibres that innervate the colon. Mean response thresholds for low threshold fibres are less than 2.5 mmHg colonic distension and mean response thresholds for high threshold fibres are greater than 30 mmHg colonic distension ; the ratio of low threshold to high threshold fibres in the rat pelvic nerve is about 3:1. The physiological roles of these two groups of afferent fibres are suggested to relate to reflex functions of the colon which are not perceived and to perceived sensations such as pressure and pain, respectively. In the present study, both low threshold and high threshold pelvic nerve fibres were studied, but there was no obvious difference between them with respect to how drugs affected their responses to colonic distension. Thus, low threshold and high threshold fibres have been grouped together in the results described below.

On the basis of conduction velocity, both C-fibres (conduction velocity less than 2.5 m/sec) and Aδ-fibres (conduction velocity greater than 2.5 m/sec, but less than 25 m/sec) were studied in the present experiments. About 60% of the sample of fibres studied were C-fibres and about 40% were Aδ-fibres. There was no obvious difference in drug effects on either C- or Aδ-fibres and they were thus grouped together in the summary of results below.

Response magnitude to colonic distension was generally increased 30 min after instillation of acetic acid into the colon ; an example is given in Figure 2. About one-half of the fibres studied were "sensitized" by intracolonic acetic acid, suggesting that

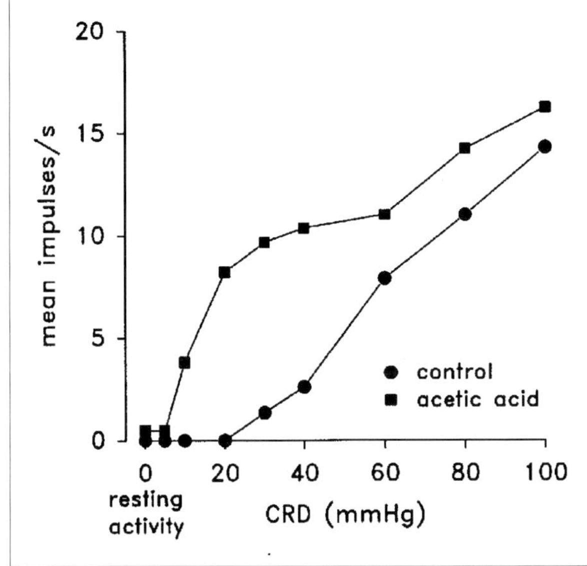

Figure 2. Sensitization of a pelvic nerve afferent fibre by intracolonic acetic acid (2.5%). The vertical axis represents the response of the fibre in mean impulses/s and the horizontal axis represents the intensity of colorectal distension (CRD) in mmHg. The stimulus-response function to CRD of this afferent fibre is shifted leftward 30 min after colonic instillation of acetic acid. The afferent fibre initially had a threshold for response to CRD of 30 mmHg, which was reduced to 10 mmHg CRD after acetic acid.

visceral afferent fibres behave like cutaneous nociceptors in response to tissue irritation or inflammation. A greater concentration of acetic acid, a longer time after intracolonic application of acetic acid, or another chemical (*e.g.*, turpentine or mustard oil) might result in a greater percentage of fibres being sensitized.

We had expected morphine to attenuate responses of pelvic nerve afferent fibres to colonic distension, but morphine was without effect on fibres recorded from either the saline-treated or acetic acid-treated colon. An example is illustrated in Figure 3. Cumulative dosages of morphine from 1-8 mg/kg were without effect on responses to 80 mmHg colonic distension. In the rat, this dose range of morphine produces significant antinociception in a wide variety of nociceptive tests. The absence of effect of morphine in these experiments suggests that morphine-produced analgesia in colorectal pain in humans is a central effect. In earlier work, lesser doses of morphine given intravenously (*e.g.*, 1-4 mg/kg) significantly attenuated both the pressor and visceromotor responses to colonic distension in unanaesthetized rats [2] and the present results lead to the conclusion that such effects were exerted in the brain and/or spinal cord. We have recently found that the intrathecal administration of either morphine or the µ-opioid receptor selective agonist DAMPGO potently and dose-dependently attenuates the pressor and visceromotor responses to colonic distension [3], confirming that activation of spinal µ-opioid receptors can modulate noxious visceral (colonic) inputs.

In contrast to the lack of effect of morphine, the κ-opioid receptor selective agonist U-50,488H dose-dependently attenuated responses of pelvic nerve afferent fibres to 80 mmHg colonic distension. An example is given in Figure 4. At the greatest dose tested (16 mg/kg), U-50,488H produced a mean attenuation of responses to about 20% of the control response to 80 mmHg colonic distension. The effects of U-50,488H were

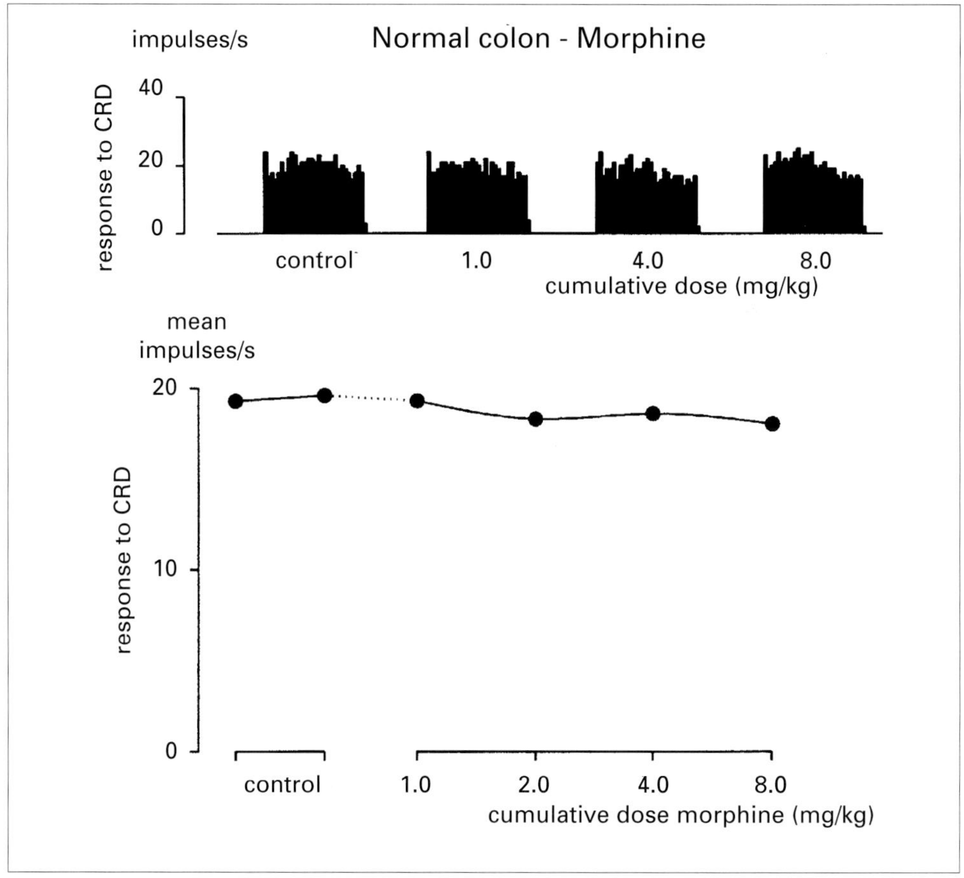

Figure 3. Lack of effect of morphine on responses of pelvic nerve afferent fibres to noxious colorectal distension (CRD). In the top panel, responses to CRD (80 mmHg) are presented as peristimulus histograms (1 s bin width) before (control) and after cumulative doses of morphine given intra-arterially. Similar data from the same afferent fibre are presented in the bottom panel, illustrating the absence of effect of morphine on pelvic nerve afferent fibre responses to noxious CRD (recorded, in this example, from the normal colon).

not reversed by a low dose of naloxone (30 µg/kg), but were reversed by a greater, total 300 µg/kg dose of naloxone. This suggests that the effects of U-50,488H were not mediated by the µ-opioid receptor, but most likely were mediated by the κ-opioid receptor. Fedotozine, which also has agonist effects at the κ-opioid receptor, similarly attenuated responses to noxious colonic distension in a dose-dependent fashion (*see* Figure 5). In comparison with U-50,488H, 16 mg/kg of fedotozine produced a mean attenuation of responses of pelvic nerve afferent fibres to 80 mmHg colonic distension to about 35% of control. Similar to U-50,488H, the effects of fedotozine were not reversed by a low dose of naloxone, but were reversed by a greater dose of naloxone that would be expected to affect κ-as well as µ-opioid receptors.

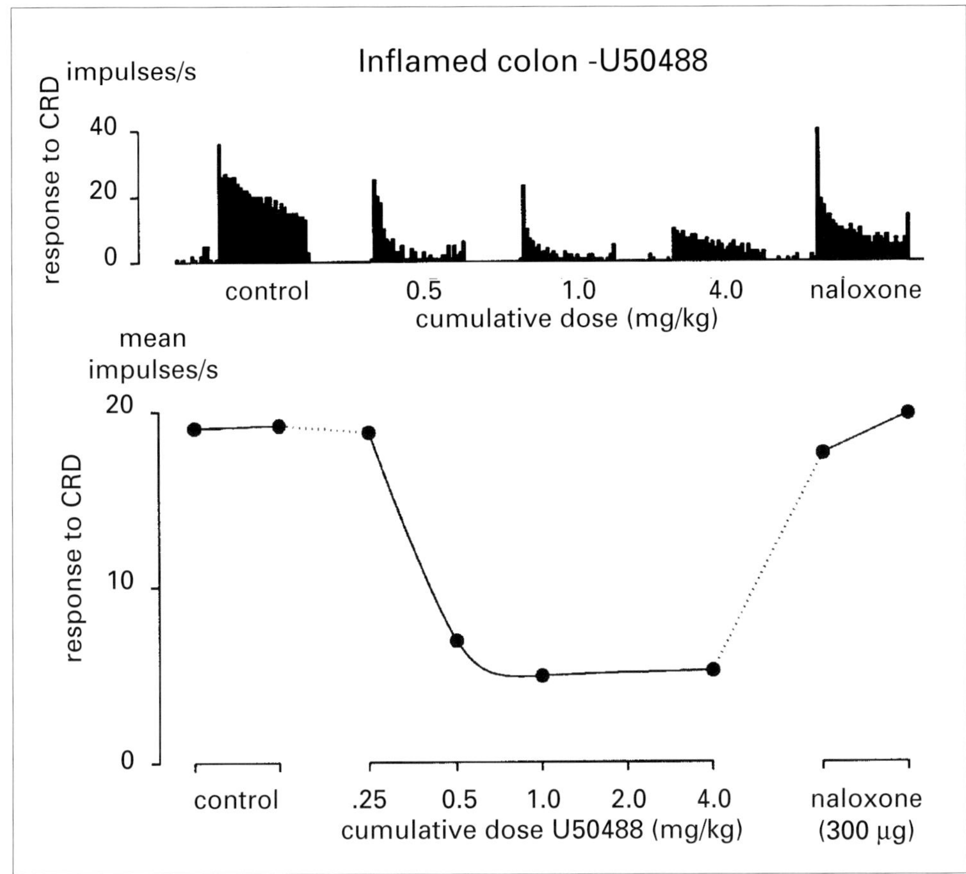

Figure 4. Effect of U-50,488H on responses of pelvic nerve afferent fibres to noxious colorectal distension (CRD). In the top panel, responses to CRD (80 mmHg) are presented as peristimulus histograms (1 s bin width) before (control) and after cumulative doses of U-50,488H given intra-arterially. Similar data from the same afferent fibre are presented in the bottom panel, illustrating the attenuation by U-50,488H on pelvic nerve afferent fibre responses to noxious CRD (recorded, in this example, from the acetic acid-treated, inflamed colon). The effect of U-50,488H in this example was reversed by a 300 µg cumulative dose of naloxone.

These effects of U-50,488H and fedotozine on responses to colonic distension in the rat are consistent with other recent reports. For example, when given into the intrathecal space in unanaesthetized rats, U-50,488H was without effect on either the pressor or visceromotor responses to noxious colorectal distension [3] ; when given intravenously, U-50,488H did attenuate the visceromotor response to colorectal distension in the same report. In barbiturate anaesthetized rats, gastrointestinal distension produces an easily quantified depressor response which is attenuated in a dose-dependent manner by U-50,488H and fedotozine when given systemically, but not when given either intracerebroventricularly or intrathecally [4, 5]. The present and previous reports thus support the conclusion that activation of peripheral, but not central κ-opioid receptors

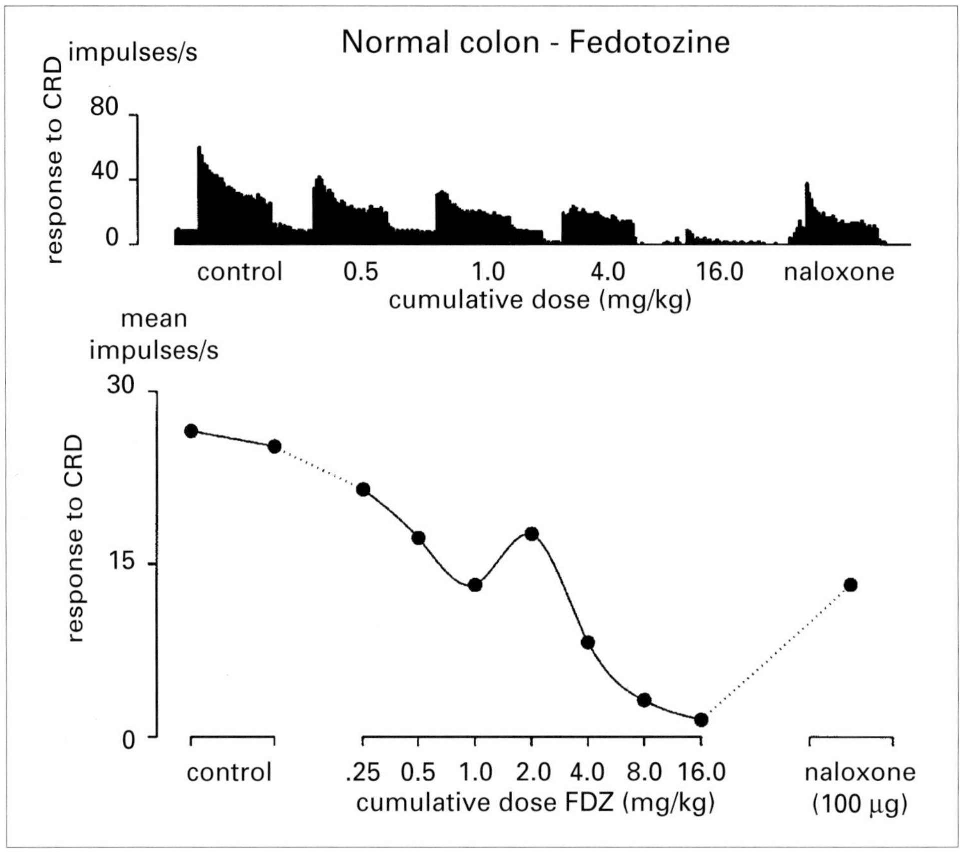

Figure 5. Effect of fedotozine on responses of pelvic nerve afferent fibres to noxious colorectal distension (CRD). In the top panel, responses to CRD (80 mmHg) are presented as peristimulus histograms (1 s bin width) before (control) and after cumulative doses of fedotozine given intra-arterially. Similar data from the same afferent fibre are presented in the bottom panel, illustrating the attenuation by fedotozine on pelvic nerve afferent fibre responses to noxious CRD (recorded, in this example, from the normal colon). The effect of fedotozine in this example was partially reversed by a 100 µg cumulative dose of naloxone.

can significantly attenuate noxious visceral inputs. This is a novel and potentially very important finding, suggesting that drugs with agonist effects at κ-opioid receptors may have a special application in the treatment of visceral pain conditions.

In conclusion, the present results document that U-50,488H and fedotozine, but not morphine, have significant and potent peripheral effects on pelvic nerve afferent fibres that innervate the colon. In the relatively limited sample of afferent fibres studied to date, we have not observed a greater effect of either U-50,488H or fedotozine on pelvic nerve fibre responses recorded from the inflamed colon. Morphine, for example, has been shown in some studies to be more potent in the presence of cutaneous inflammation and one might expect that U-50,488H or fedotozine would also show a left-shifted dose-response function in the presence of colonic inflammation. The model studied here, however, does not adequately reproduce the natural condition, where inflammation or colonic hypersensitivity may be of rather long standing. We studied drug effects on responses to colonic distension only 30 min after intracolonic instillation of acetic acid. Another model of inflammation which more closely approximates the human condition may reveal a relatively greater effect of U-50,488H or fedotozine, a condition that we plan to investigate in the future.

References

1. Sengupta JN, Gebhart GF. Characterization of mechanosensitive pelvic nerve afferent fibres innervating the colon of the rat. *J Neurophysiol* 1994 ; 71 : 2046-60.
2. Ness TJ, Gebhart GF. Colorectal distension as a noxious visceral stimulus: physiological and pharmacological characterization of pseudoaffective reflexes in the rat. *Brain Res* 1988 ; 450 : 153-69.
3. Danzebrink R, Green S, Gebhart GF. Spinal mu and delta, but not kappa, opioid receptor agonists attenuate responses to noxious colorectal distension in the rat. *Pain* 1995 ; in press.
4. Diop L, Riviere PJM, Pascaud X, Dassaud M, Junien JL. Role of vagal afferents in the antinociception produced by morphine and U-50,488H in the colonic pain reflex in rat. *Eur J Pharmacol* 1994 ; 257 : 181-7.
5. Diop L, Riviere PJM, Pascaud X, Junien JL. Antinociceptive effect of fedotozine on the duodenal pain reflex in rat. *Eur J Pharmacol* 1994 ; 271 : 65-71.

Sensitive gastrointestinal disorders. J.P. Galmiche, B. Fraitag.
John Libbey Eurotext, Paris © 1995, pp. 73-76

9

Effect of fedotozine on gastric visceral nociception in healthy subjects

B. COFFIN, M. LÉMANN**, B. FRAITAG***, R. JIAN***

** INSERM U 290, Hôpital Saint-Lazare, Paris, France.*
*** Service de Gastroentérologie, Hôpital Saint-Louis, Paris, France.*
**** Institut de Recherche Jouveinal, Fresnes, France.*

Patients with functional dyspepsia exhibit an increased sensitivity to gastric distension, but no drug is available to specifically reverse this abnormality. Fedotozine has been shown to have anti-nociceptive activity in several experimental animal models.

We thus conducted three series of experiments in healthy volunteers to investigate the effect of fedotozine on gastric sensitivity. The results of the two series of experiments testing the effect of fedotozine on discomfort threshold during gastric distension were pooled and globally analysed. These experiments included 27 healthy subjects randomized to receive either fedotozine (30 mg t.i.d.), or a placebo during seven days. Gastric distensions were performed at day 7 while the subject received the last tablet of his allocated treatment. In these experiments, we also tested in 11 volunteers the effect of fedotozine on post-prandial gastric tone and in 16 volunteers the effect of fedotozine on peripheral sensitivity. Finally, in a third series of experiments, including 10 healthy subjects, the effect of fedotozine on gastric sensitivity was assessed by a reflexologic technique.

Gastric distension tests

The distensions were performed with an electronic barostat, the balloon of the barostat being placed in the proximal stomach. Each distension was sustained during 2 minutes and followed by a 5-minute rest period. We performed firstly isobaric distensions with 2 mgHg increment until 20 mgHg or discomfort threshold was reached, and thereafter isovolumic distensions with 200 ml increment until 1,000 ml or until discomfort threshold. Sensations were scored by a verbal questionnaire, and we defined prospectively the sensation of discomfort at an intense and sustained sensation (Figure 1).

During isobaric distensions, fedotozine increased significantly both the threshold pressure and the threshold volume at which the sensation of discomfort was first perceived by the volunteers. During isovolumic distension, the same tendency was observed, but a carry-over did not allow statistical evaluation of the action of

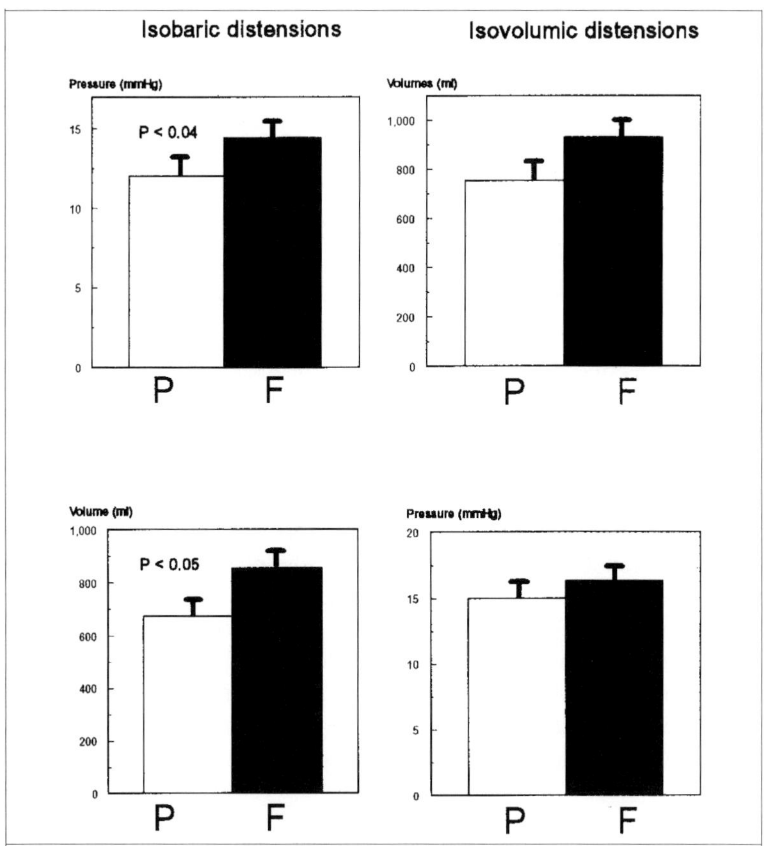

Figure 1. Effect of fedotozine on thresholds for discomfort during isobaric and isovolumic gastric distensions. P : placebo, F: fedotozine.

fedotozine. Gastric compliance, measured during these experiments, was not affected by fedotozine.

Post-prandial tone measurement

As previously described, the meal induced a marked and prolonged relaxation of the stomach, evidenced by the increase in the volume of the balloon of the barostat. In contrast, fedotozine did not significantly modify the magnitude or the kinetic of this gastric relaxation.

Cold-stress experiments

We tested the effect of fedotozine on somatic sensitivity by performing a cold stress. For this, the temperature of the non-dominant hand of the subject was changed from 37° to 4° and thereafter the reversed experiment was performed. The nociceptive sensations, evaluated by a visual analog scale, were not significantly affected by fedotozine.

Reflexologic experiments

The reflexologic technique used involves a nociceptive cutaneous muscular reflex (R III reflex) continuously elicited by electrical stimulation of the sural nerve. Gastric distension inhibits this reflex, and we have shown in a recently published paper, that this inhibition correlates both with the level of the distension — here the pressure within the bag of the barostat — and the sensation perceived by the subject and elicited by the distension [1]. In this double-blind controlled randomized study, two sequences were performed with a one-week washout period : one with fedotozine and the other with placebo. On each sequence, we performed a basal evaluation without drug and a therapeutic evaluation at day 7 while the subject received his allocated treatment. R III reflex was continuously stimulated, and a gastric distension of 1,000 ml was performed. During the two basal evaluations (without drug), the gastric distension inhibited R III reflex. This inhibition was intense (more than 50% of the pre-distension intensity) and sustained during the 3 minutes of the distension period. The placebo did not significantly modify this response. Fedotozine significantly decreased the inhibition, as compared to placebo, but this effect was only significant during the first minute of distension (Figure 2).

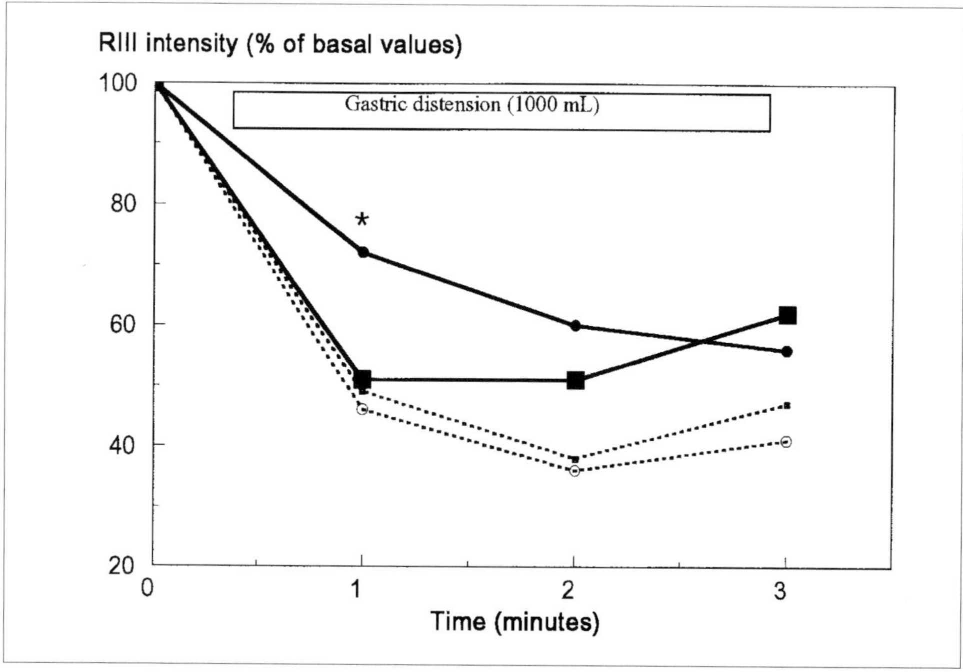

Figure 2. Effect of fedotozine on R III reflex intensity expressed as percentages of predistension values. Dotted lines depicted experiments performed before treatment, black squares experiments performed on placebo, and black circles experiments performed on fedotozine.
* : p<0.05 *vs* placebo.

Conclusion

We showed that fedotozine increased significantly the threshold pressure at which gastric discomfort is perceived by healthy subjects while it does not affect gastric compliance, post-prandial tone and somatic sensitivity. Fedotozine also decreases the inhibition of the R III reflex, a phenomenon closely related to visceral nociception, during the first minute of a 3 minute gastric distension period. These results suggest that fedotozine decreases gastric sensitivity to distension, an effect which may be related to an action on afferent visceral pathways. Under the present experimental conditions, this effect seems to be limited to the indication of the visceral stimulation.

Reference

1. Bouhassira D, Chollet R, Coffin B, Lémann M, Le Bars D, Willer JC, Jian R. Inhibition of a somatic nociceptive reflex by gastric distension in humans. *Gastroenterology* 1994 ; 107 : 985-92.

Sensitive gastrointestinal disorders. J.P. Galmiche, B. Fraitag.
John Libbey Eurotext, Paris © 1995, pp. 77-79

10

Intestinal sensitivity in healthy volunteers : a pilot study of the action of fedotozine

CH. KREISS*, R. FRASER*, J. BOROVICKA*, K. ASAL*, W. SCHWIZER*,
A. BISCHOF-DELALOYE*, N. READ**, J.L. ABITBOL***, A.L. BLUM****, M. FRIED*

* Policlinique Médicale Universitaire, 1005 Lausanne, Switzerland.
** University Hospital of Sheffield, UK.
*** Institut de Recherche Jouveinal, Fresnes, France.
**** Centre Hospitalier Universitaire Vaudois, Lausanne, Switzerland.

Fedotozine is a peripheral κ-receptor agonist which has been suggested to affect gastrointestinal sensitivity, including an action on sensory feedback mechanisms arising from the small intestine. Intraduodenal infusion of lipids slows gastric emptying by a suppression of antral motility and stimulation of pyloric contractions [1]. Thus the intraduodenal infusion of lipids constitutes a model to investigate small intestinal feedback mechanisms.

The aim of this pilot study was to investigate whether fedotozine abolishes the delay of gastric emptying induced by an intraduodenal infusion of fat and to find the appropriate dose of fedotozine eliciting this effect. The following experimental protocol was employed : after an overnight fast, an enteric feeding tube was positioned in the distal duodenum for the infusion of Intralipid® 10%. Subsequently, a test meal consisting of a pancake (340 kcal) labelled with 500 mCi 99mTc sulphur colloid and 500 ml dextrose 10% was given. Gastric emptying was measured for 150 min in a sitting position using a dual-headed gamma-camera and calculating the geometric mean of the anterior and posterior images. The experiments were performed at the same time of the day in all subjects. Thirty minutes after start of gastric emptying, the intraduodenal lipid infusion was administered at 1 ml/min for 30 min through the feeding tube. Two experiments were performed in a single-blind crossover design. Two healthy volunteers were studied after i.v. infusion of fedotozine 12.5 mg and placebo and two others were studied after i.v. infusion of fedotozine 12.5 mg and 50 mg. The infusion was started directly after meal ingestion and was continued for 60 to 80 min.

The gastric emptying curve was divided into three parts : before, during and after duodenal lipid infusion and the slopes of linear regression were calculated for these three periods. The results are shown in Table I. Intralipid markedly slowed gastric emptying in all volunteers. Gastric emptying accelerated after the end of the lipid infusion. The delay of gastric emptying was abolished by fedotozine and this effect was more pronounced at the dose of 50 mg as compared to 12.5 mg. An example in one volunteer, who received 12.5 mg and 50 mg, is shown in Figure 1. Whereas Intralipid® inhibited gastric emptying during the infusion of 12.5 mg of fedotozine, the dose of 50 mg resulted in an unaltered gastric emptying curve despite the intraduodenal lipid infusion.

Table I. Slopes of linear regression for the three parts of the experiments : part BL (beginning of gastric emptying until start of duodenal lipid infusion), part IL (during duodenal lipid infusion) and PL (end of IL until end of measurement).

Volunteer	Treatment	Periods of experiment		
		BL	IL	PL
1	Placebo	-0.3	0.1	-0.4
	Fz 12.5 mg	-0.2	-0.2	-0.5
2	Placebo	-0.3	-0.2	-0.2
	Fz 12.5 mg	-0.2	-0.2	-0.1
3	Fz 12.5 mg	-0.1	-0.3	-0.5
	Fz 50 mg	-0.3	-0.4	-0.7
4	Fz 12.5 mg	-0.5	-0.5	-0.6
	Fz 50 mg	-0.7	-0.6	-0.5

In conclusion, the delay of gastric emptying caused by the intraduodenal infusion of Intralipid® 10% was abolished by fedotozine and this effect is more pronounced at the dose of 50 mg as compared to 12.5 mg. Thus, this pilot study has shown that i.v. fedotozine inhibits the activation of fat-dependent intestinal feedback mechanisms regulating gastric emptying in humans.

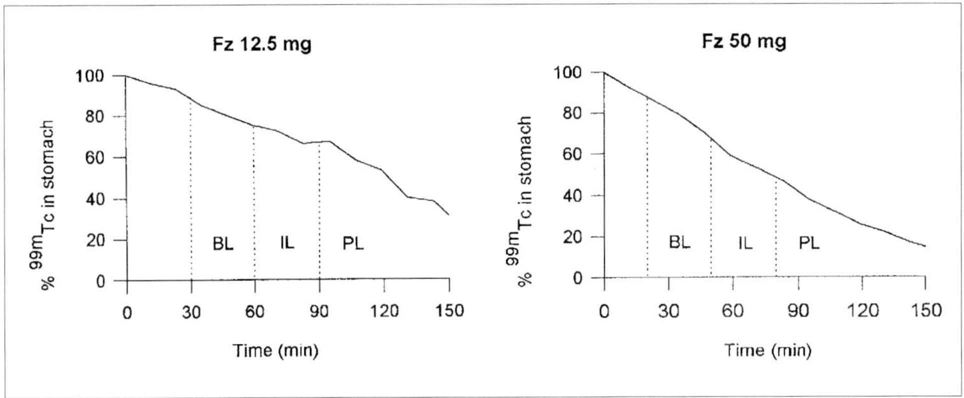

Figure 1. Comparison of fedotozine 12.5 mg and 50 mg in one volunteer : gastric emptying during the three parts of the experiment : part BL (beginning of gastric emptying until start of duodenal lipid infusion), part IL (during duodenal lipid infusion) and PL (end of IL until end of measurement).

Reference

1. Heddle R, Collins PJ, Dent J, Horowitz M, Read NW, Chatterton B, Houghton A. Motor mechanisms associated with slowing of the gastric emptying of a solid meal by an intraduodenal lipid infusion. *J Gastroenterol Hepatol* 1989 ; 4 : 437-47.

Sensitive gastrointestinal disorders. J.P. Galmiche, B. Fraitag
John Libbey Eurotext, Paris © 1995, pp. 81- 88.

11

The effect of sleep deprivation on gastric emptying and food intake in healthy volunteers : action of fedotozine

N.W. READ

Centre for Human Nutrition, Northern General Hospital, Sheffield, UK.

Short periods of total sleep deprivation are associated with decreased wakefullness, the onset of negative mood changes and by incoherent visual misperception and temporal and cognitive disorientation [1-5]. These psychological changes are associated with EEG changes suggestive of cortical irritability. Previous studies carried out in our laboratory have shown that a period of sleep deprivation can increase the sensitivity of the rectum to mechanical distension [6] and also reduce the consumption of food [7], increasing the feelings of satiety when smaller amounts have been consumed. These observations suggest that sleep deprivation may provide a useful means of investigating the effects of cortical irritability on gastrointestinal function.

Fedotozine is an opioid analogue that acts on κ-receptors in the gastrointestinal tract to reverse the physiological effects of stress. Studies carried out in dogs have shown that oral fedotozine can reverse the increases in plasma cortisol and the delays in gastric emptying induced by acoustic stress [8] ; both of these effects can be blocked by cutting the vagus. This raises the possibility that fedotozine may be helpful in treating functional diseases that have a strong association with psychosocial stress. The aim of the study was to investigate whether sleep deprivation could alter gastric emptying and food intake in normal volunteers and to determine whether these changes could be inhibited by prior administration of fedotozine.

Material and methods

Subjects

There were 20 normal male volunteers (aged 21 to 34 ; median age 23) who had no history of bowel disease. None of the subjects were regular smokers or consumed greater than 14 units alcohol a week. All had a normal weight for their height and age. All the subjects had a full medical examination and underwent haematological and biochemical screening tests prior to entry to the study. The results were normal in every case.

Each of the subjects was fully informed as to the nature and aims of the study and written consent was obtained before entry to the study. The protocol was approved by the Ethical Committee of the Northern General Hospital, Sheffield.

Protocol

The protocol is illustrated in Figure 1. Baseline measurements of gastric emptying were performed up to 7 days before randomisation (D-6 to D0). Subjects were then randomised on D0 to 2 parallel groups of 10 subjects, who received either fedotozine one 30 mg tablet t.i.d. or placebo one tablet three times a day for (D1 to D5) or an identical placebo tablet three times a day for the same period of time. Both the subjects and the investigators were blind as to the treatment each subject received.

Subjects fasted from 6 pm on the evening of day 3 were admitted to the investigation unit at 8 am on day 4 of the study and remained awake under constant supervision throughout the study period which ended at 8.15 pm on day 5. The subjects were free

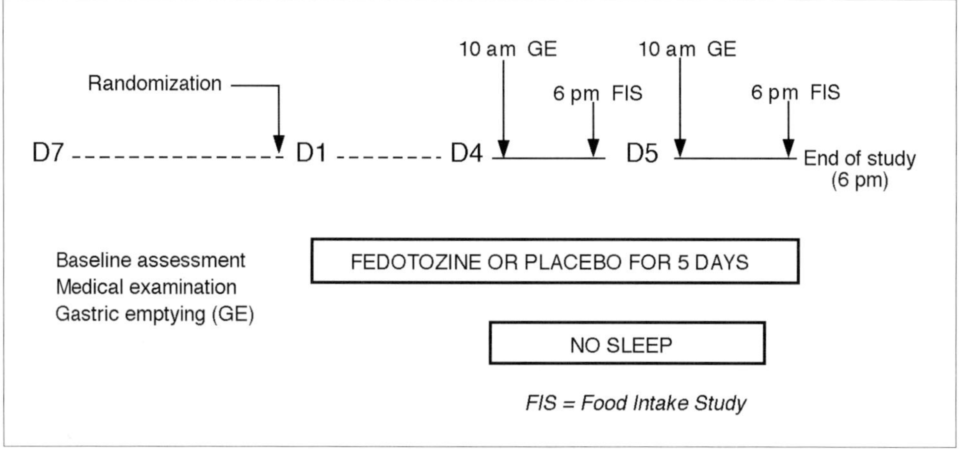

Figure 1. Study design.

to read, watch television or play boardgames. The pattern of meal consumption on days 4 and 5 was identical. Each subject consumed a high fat soup at 10 am for the gastric emptying study, a standard lunch (1000 Kcal) at 1.30 pm, the test meal for the food intakes study at 6 pm and a light snack (100 Kcal) at 11.30 pm. Fluids were unrestricted (orange juice or water) but the amounts consumed were recorded. Alcohol and tobacco were prohibited for both groups throughout the study period.

Gastric emptying

Gastric emptying was measured during the baseline period before randomisation and at 10 am on study days 4 and 5. The subjects fasted for 10 hours before each study. The subjects sat vertically against a posteriorly positioned gamma camera (modes 1201 Pho/Gamma scintillation camera, Nuclear-Chicago, Europa NV, Amsterdam, the Netherlands). The subjects then consumed within 2 minutes 300 ml of radiolabelled (1.89 MBq 99m Technetium-Tin colloid) beef consomme (Campbell Grovery Products, Kings Lynn, Norfolk) in which had been blended 30 g margerine (SUMA Sunflower Margarine, Halifax, West Yorks). The composition of these meals was 33 g fat, 1.2 g carbohydrates, 4.2 g protein. Previous studies have shown that the fat in the soup did not separate out after *in vitro* incubation with 0.1M Hydrochloric acid for 3 hours [9].

As soon as the liquid meals was consumed, images of the distribution of the radioactivity in the abdominal cavity were collected over consecutive 2 minute periods for the first 45 frames, and over consecutive 5 minute periods for the next 22 frames. The total period of data collecion was 200 minutes. At the end of the study, a further 1.89 MBq 99m Technetium-Tin colloid in 150 ml water was given orally and a left lateral image of the stomach obtained by the posteriorly positioned gamma camera can be corrected for tissue attenuation caused by the isotope moving away from the camera as the meal empties [10, 11].

Analysis of the gamma camera records proceeded in the following manner. The position of the stomach was identified from the images obtained during the first 10 minutes of the study and outlined using a cursor. The computer then extracted the counts from the region of interest, corrected them for decay and tissue attenuation and expressed them as a percentage of the counts obtained in the gastric region immediately after ingestion of the meal. These figures were then used to construct profiles of the proportion of counts in the stomach throughout the study. The gastric emptying profiles were then analysed to yield values for : (i) the time taken for half the isotope to empty from the sotmach (t1/2) ; (ii) the percentage of isotope remaining in the stomach 100 minutes after ingestion.

Eating behaviour : test meal

At 6 pm on each study day (D4 and D5), the subjects were presented with an appetising meal, preselected from a menu and prepared in excess of what they would normally be expected to eat. Orange squash was provided to drink and subjects were invited to consume as much food and squash as they wished to comfort. The amount of food and drink consumed and the time taken to complete the meal were recorded and from these figures, values for the energy intake, the rates of eating and drinking and the time taken to complete the meal were measured.

Statistical analysis

Comparability of the treatment groups
The Student's test for independent samples (two tailed test) was used to compare the means of the two groups (placebo and fedotozine) for demographic characteristics, sleeping habits, half-emptying time and percentage remaining in the stomach at 100 minutes.

Treatment effect
The change over time on treatment was compared between the two treatment groups by a two way analysis of variance (treatment x time) with repeated measurements over time.

An intergroup analysis has been performed using a one way analysis of variance (time factor) with repeated measurements over time.

Contrasts *versus* baseline have been tested. According to the protocol, a comparison of the two groups on the variation between day 3 and day 4 was performed.

The type I error (α) allowed for these analyses was 5%

Results

Baseline measures

There were no significant differences between the two groups of volunteers in the numbers of hours slept on the night before sleep deprivation or the normal average hours slept per night. Neither were there any significant differences in the baseline measurements of gastric emptying, although it was notable that the average half time for gastric emptying in the fedotozine group was 30 minutes slower than that in the placebo group (Table I).

Effect of sleep deprivation

Sleep deprivation increased the scores for drowsiness in both groups of volunteers, but did not affect scores for calmness or excitement, happiness or sadness. Both groups

Table I. Effect of sleep deprivation on gastric emptying (results expressed as half emptying time in minutes)..

	Baseline	Day 4	Day 5	Δ D5-D4
Placebo n = 10	77 ± 18	61 ± 15	101 ± 17 *p = 0.009*	40 ±7
Fedotozine n = 10	47 ± 5	49 ± 7	71 ± 14 *p = 0.126*	22 ± 14

mean ± SEM ; *p* value comparing day 4 and day 5

of subjects thought they had eaten less food after sleep deprivation and expressed a reduced satiety to eat.

Gastric emptying

Following the period of sleep deprivation there was a significant delay in gastric emptying in the placebo group, assessed by both the half emptying time and the percentage of isotope remaining at 100 minutes. There was also a delay in gastric emptying in the fedotozine group but this did not achieve statistical significance (Figure 2). Comparison of the differences before and after sleep deprivation for the two groups

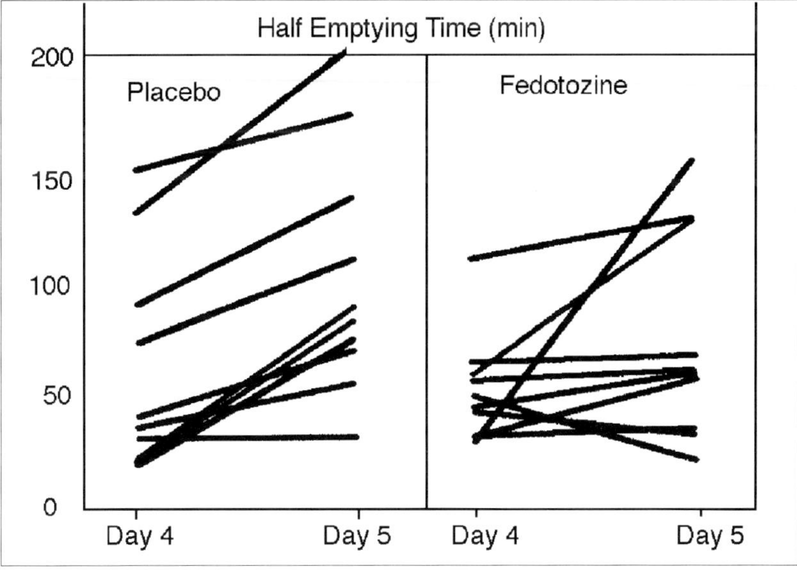

Figure 2. Results of gastric emptying ; results are expressed as half emptying time (individual data). Day 4: before and day 5: after sleep deprivation.

showed no significant effect of fedotozine on the changes induced by sleep deprivation (Table I).

Food intake

The results of the food intake studies showed significant reductions in the total calorie intake and total food weight in both the placebo and fedotozine groups.

The time taken to eat the meals was unchanged in both groups.

The results did not show any significant differences in the magnitude of the change following sleep deprivation between the two groups (Table II).

Table II. Effects of sleep deprivation and fedotozine on food intake.

	Regimens	Day 4	Day 5	Δ D5-D4
Calories	Placebo n = 10	2064 ± 259	1747 ± 229 *p = 0.014*	-317 ± 80
(kcal)	Fedotozine n = 10	1855 ± 142	1606 ± 149 *p = 0.006*	-248 ± 51
Food Weight	Placebo n = 10	1085 ± 81	865 ± 71 *p = 0.006*	-220 ± 52
(grams)	Fedotozine n = 10	972 ± 62	859 ± 65 *p = 0.011*	-113 ± 29

mean ± SEM ; *p* values comparing day 4 and day 5

Discussion

The results of this study indicate that, in healthy volunteers, a period of total sleep deprivation of 24 hours can delay emptying of a lipid rich meal from the stomach, and reduce food intake in healthy volunteers. Moreover, fedotozine may prevent, at least partially, this delay.

How might sleep deprivation induce these changes ? Short periods of total sleep deprivation are not associated with any significant changes in stress related hormones such as catecholamines [12] or cortisol [13], nor in any of the physiological indices of autonomic nervous activity [12, 14, 15]. The principle effects of short periods of total sleep deprivation in humans are seen at the cerebral level with altered cognition [16], negative mood changes [17], and abnormalities in the EEG [18]. These changes suggest the effect is more one of cerebral depression than of arousal as seen in acute stress. The mechanism by which the changes observed in this study came about seems therefore more likely to be centrally mediated.

The reason for the delay in gastric emptying seen in the placebo group is not entirely certain but may relate to an increased sensitivity of the duodenum to the presence of lipid in the meal. An increase in gastrointestinal sensitivity was also observed in a previous study, in which sleep deprivation increased the sensitivity of the rectum to mechanical distension [6].

References

1. Bohlin G, Kjellberg A. Self reported arousal during sleep derivation and its relation to performance and physiological variables. *Scand J Physiol* 1973 ; 14 : 78-86.
2. Naitoh P. Chronopsychological approach for optimizing human performance. In: Brown FM, Graeber RC, eds. *Rhythmic aspects of behaviour*. Hillsdale: NJ Lawrence Erlbaum, 1982 : 110-125.
3. Mikulincer M, Babkoff H, Caspy T, Sing H. The effects of 72 hours sleep loss on psychological variables. *Br J Psychol* 1989 ; 80 : 145-62.
4. Cutler MR, Cohen HB. The effect of one night's sleep loss on mood and memory in normal subjects. *Comp Psychiatry* 1979 ; 20 : 61-6.
5. Horne JA. A review of the biological effects of total sleep deprivation in man. *Biol Psychol* 1978 ; 7 : 55-102.
6. Bergin AJ, Read NW. The effects of sleep deprivation on rectal sensitivity in healthy volunteers. *Eur J Gastroenterol Hepatol* 1993 ; 5 : 527-32.
7. Bergin AJ, Daly J, Sepple CP, French S, Read NW. The effect of sleep deprivation on food intake and satiety in healthy male volunteers (submitted for publication).
8. Buéno L, Gué M, Fargeas M, Alvinerne M, Furien JL, Fiaromonti J. Vagally medicated inhibition of acoustic stress involved cortisol release by orally administered κ–opioid substances in dogs. *Endocrinology* ; 124 : 1788-93.
9. Houghton LA, Mangnall YF, Read NW. Effects of incorporating fat into a liquid test meal on the relation between intragastric distribution and gastric emptying in human volunteers. *Gut* 1990 ; 31 : 1226-9.
10. Collins PJ, Horowitz M, Cook DJ, Harding PE, Shearman DJC. Gastric emptying in normal subjects - a reproducible technique using a simple scintillation counter and a computer system. *Gut* 1983 ; 24 : 1117-25.
11. Collins PJ, Horowitz M, Shearman DJC, Chatterton BE. Correction for tissue attenuation in radionuclide gastric emptying studies : a comparison of a lateral image method and a geometric mean method. *Br J Radiol* 1984 ; 57 : 689-95.
12. Fiorica V, Higgins EA, Iampietro PF, Lategola MT, Davies AW. Physiological responses of men during sleep deprivation. *J Appl Physiol* 1968 ; 24 : 167-76.
13. Bliss EL, Clark LD, West CD. Studies of sleep deprivation : relationship to schizophrenia. *Arch Neurol Psychiatry* 1959 ; 81 : 348-59.
14. Corcoran DWJ. Changes in heart rate and performance as a result as a loss of sleep. *Br J Psychol* 1964 ; 55 : 307-15.

15. Bruce LC. Some observations upon the general blood pressures in sleeplessness and sleep. *Scott Med Surg J* 1900 ; 7 : 109-17.
16. French SJ, Read NW. The effect of lipid and viscous polysaccharide on gastric emptying and feelings of hunger. *Gut* 1992 ; 33 (suppl.) : S54 (abstract).
17. Wyatt S, Marriot R. Night work and shift changes. *Br J Industr Med* 1953 ; 10 : 164-72.
18. Hakkinen S. Adaptability to shift work. In : Swensonn A, ed. *Night and shift work*. Stockholm, Studia laboris et salutis ; 1969 ; 4 : 68-80.

Third session

Fedotozine contribution to drug therapy

Sensitive gastrointestinal disorders. J.P. Galmiche, B. Fraitag.
John Libbey Eurotext, Paris © 1995, pp. 91-98

12

Update on the clinical development of fedotozine in functional dyspepsia and irritable bowel syndrome*

B. FRAITAG

Institut de Recherche Jouveinal, Fresnes, France.

The development plan of fedotozine in functional dyspepsia (FD) and irritable bowel syndrome (IBS) included a phase I which was common to both indications and then a very similar design in either indication, *i.e.* a dose-finding phase II including a small pilot phase II-A study, followed by a larger phase II-B dose range study; having the therapeutic dose derived from phase II, phase III was undertaken, including two studies *versus* placebo in each indication, plus two studies *versus* an active comparator in dyspepsia. In the IBS, it is indeed well accepted that no reference compound exists at the moment, so that only studies *versus* placebo were carried out ; in addition, studies common to both indications were performed, including a one year safety study in over 400 patients, a safety study in the elderly over 75 years of age.

---

* Some of the trials reported in this review are not yet published. (Data on file, Institut de Recherche Jouveinal.)

Methods

This was mainly a European development with further studies conducted outside Europe, *e.g.* in Canada. Each study was carried out in a single language. From phase II-B on, the trials were large and multicentre with 150 to 300 patients. The active treatment period has always been 6 weeks in parallel groups and the protocols were similar, allowing a global analysis of results. Good Clinical Practice standards were demanded in each study with a quality control.

The definitions and assessment criteria used in FD and IBS are listed on Table I. The symptoms which define dyspepsia are all primarily post-prandial, and in IBS, the main symptom was lower abdominal pain or discomfort plus other symptoms among the so-called Manning's criteria. The main criterion has always been derived from the patient's own assessment of his/her global symptomatology in dyspepsia or of his/her lower abdominal pain in IBS. In addition, safety has been studied, as well as quality of life, which may be very relevant to these functional conditions.

The main criterion of efficacy has been derived from a daily assessment of his/her symptoms by the patient on diary cards. An example is shown on Figure 1.

Table I. Functional dyspepsia and irritable bowel syndrome: inclusion and assessment criteria.

	Functional dyspepsia	Irritable bowel syndrome
- Symptoms (*patient*/investigator)	- *Global symptomatology*	*Lower abdominal pain*
	- Epigastric pain	- + other symptoms among Manning's criteria
	- Feeling of slow digestion	
	- Inability to finish a normal meal	
	- Epigastric fullness/bloating	
	- Nausea/vomiting	
	(all primarily post-prandial)	
- Quality of life	X	X
- Safety	X	X

Main criteria are indicated in italic.

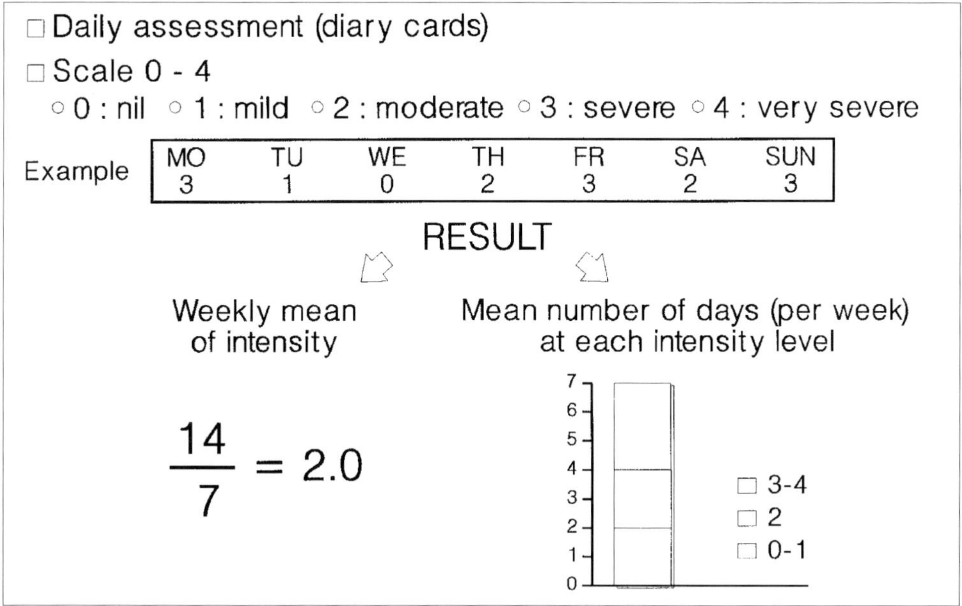

Figure 1. Main criterion of efficacy in dyspepsia and irritable bowel syndrome : two ways expression of the data from the diary cards.

Efficacy

In dyspepsia, phase II-A included a small pilot study with 9, 18, 70, 210 mg t.i.d. of fedotozine *versus* placebo, which showed that 18 and 70 mg were better than placebo. So the larger phase II-B study was carried out with the doses of 10, 30, 70 mg t.i.d. *versus* placebo. The doses of 30 and 70 mg t.i.d. were both better than placebo, but there was no significant difference between 30 and 70 mg so that 30 mg t.i.d was considered the therapeutic dose [1].

The results of this phase II-B study regarding the main assessment criterion appear on Table II.

Table II. Results of phase II-B study in patients with functional dyspepsia. Results are expressed as mean symptom score (mean ± SD) during four different periods (P_1 = run-in, P_2 = week 1-2, P_3 = week 3-4 and P_4 = week 5-6).

	Number of patients	P_1	P_2	P_3	P_4
Placebo	41	1.88 ± 1.26	1.54 ± 1.18	1.38 ± 1.21	1.33 ± 1.22
Fedotozine 10 mg	32	2.06 ± 1.16	1.63 ± 1.23	1.43 ± 1.19	1.29 ± 1.21
Fedotozine 30 mg	33	2.17 ± 0.98[a]	1.45 ± 1.23[a]	1.05 ± 1.13[a]	0.93 ± 1.05[a]
Fedotozine 70 mg	25	1.87 ± 0.81[b]	1.18 ± 0.84[b]	0.87 ± 0.69[b]	0.67 ± 0.54[b]

a. p = 0.0013   Fedotozine 30 mg *versus* placebo (linear trend) - improvement
b. p = 0.0185   Fedotozine 70 mg *versus* placebo (linear trend) - improvement

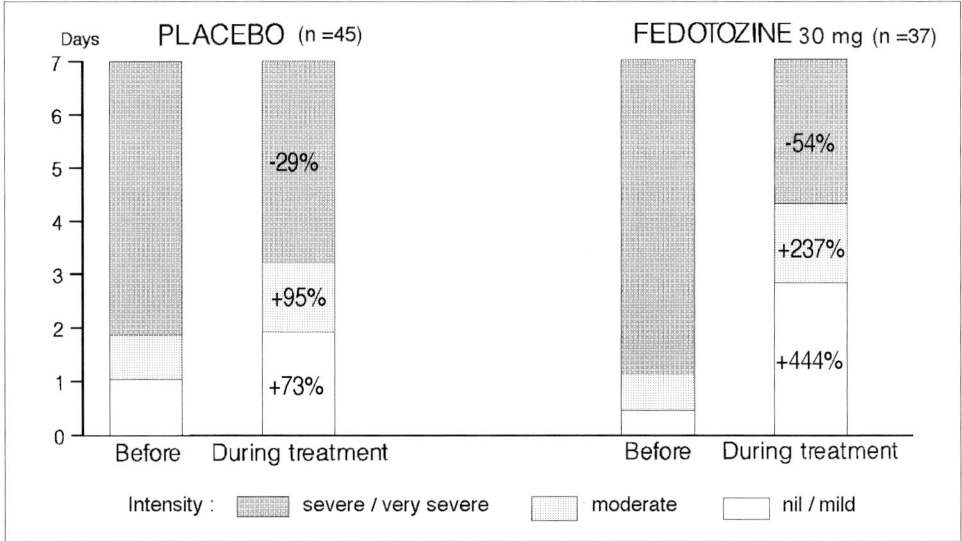

Figure 2. Dose-range study in dyspepsia : number of days (per week) of the symptomatology at each intensity level before and during treatment. Symptomatology = most severe symptom of the day. Treatment effect : p= 0.034.

The other way of expressing the same results is shown on Figure 2. The mean number of days at intensity nil or mild rose by 73% on placebo and 444% on fedotozine. In the same study, a number of individual symptoms were also significantly improved on 30 and/or 70 mg of fedotozine, including fullness, bloating, belching marginally, nausea and epigastric pain. The first phase III study was a multicenter trial *versus* placebo carried out in France. In this study, there was a significant improvement *versus* placebo on fedotozine in the per-protocol population [2]. The other way of expressing the same results shows an increase of 36% of the days with intensity nil or mild on placebo, 67% on fedotozine (Figure 3).

The next study *versus* placebo was carried out in the United Kingdom and Ireland (*see* next chapter). Another phase III study *versus* metoclopramide was carried out in France and showed that fedotozine 30 mg t.i.d. and metoclopramide 10 mg t.i.d. brought about an equivalent improvement on the main criterion in the intention-to-treat analysis [3]. It may be of interest that the safety of the two compounds was different : the number of central nervous system related side effects was higher on metoclopramide than on fedotozine, as expected.

An other study *versus* an active comparator was carried out in the Netherlands *versus* cisapride 5 mg t.i.d., and showed a significant equivalence between the two compounds regarding the main criterion in the intention-to-treat analysis. The global analysis of all studies including a 30 mg t.i.d. group and a placebo group demonstrated a significant treatment effect of fedotozine. The number of days at intensity nil or mild rose by 61%

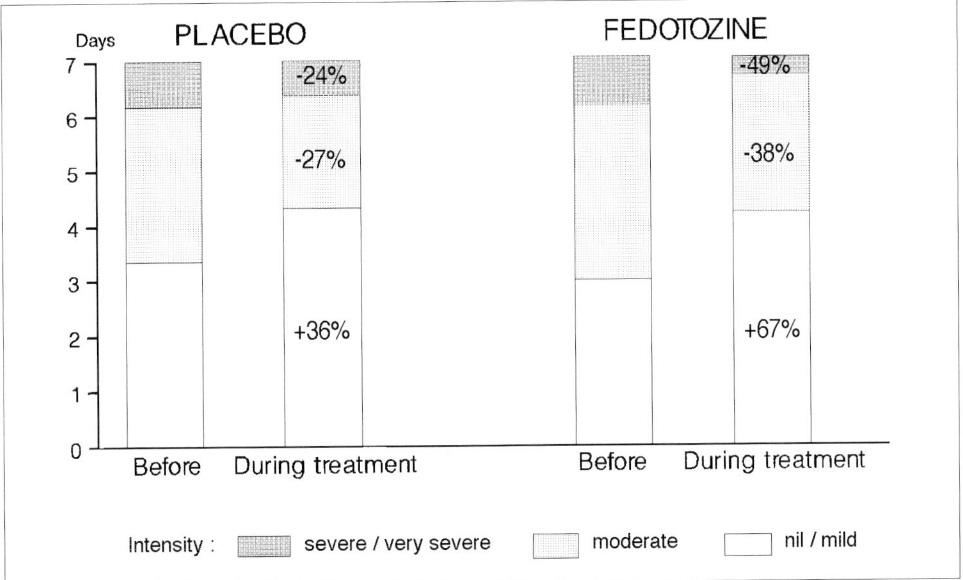

Figure 3. Phase III study *vs* placebo in dyspepsia (France) : number of days (per week) of the overall intensity of dyspepsia symptoms at each intensity level before and during treatment (analysis per protocol n =163). The effect of treatment was statistically significant (p = 0.017).

on placebo and by 116% on fedotozine. In the same global analysis, a number of symptoms were also significantly improved in the intention-to-treat analysis, including epigastric pain, nausea or vomiting, fullness, bloating and marginally the feeling of "slow digestion".

In irritable bowel syndrome, virtually the same development plan was followed with an initial small phase II-A study comparing the doses of 9, 35, 90, 140 and 210 mg t.i.d. after a placebo. This study showed that 9 and 35 mg t.i.d. of fedotozine appeared to be better than placebo, hence the doses tested in the larger phase II-B study : 3.5, 15, 30 mg t.i.d. *versus* a placebo in four parallel groups. In the latter study, 30 mg appeared to be better than placebo [4]. Thus, the therapeutic dose in IBS appeared to be also 30 mg t.i.d. (*see* chapter 14).

A one-year open study was aiming particularly at safety, but in the same study, the patients were asked to rate their satisfaction at 3, 6, 9 and 12 months, and it may be of interest that the number of patients recording an improvement at 12 months was 87.5%. The proportion of patients reporting a total disappearance of symptoms increased over the twelve months of the study. Though no firm conclusion about efficacy can be drawn from this open study, it is noteworthy to mention that 423 out of 628 patients were still followed at twelve months (Figure 4).

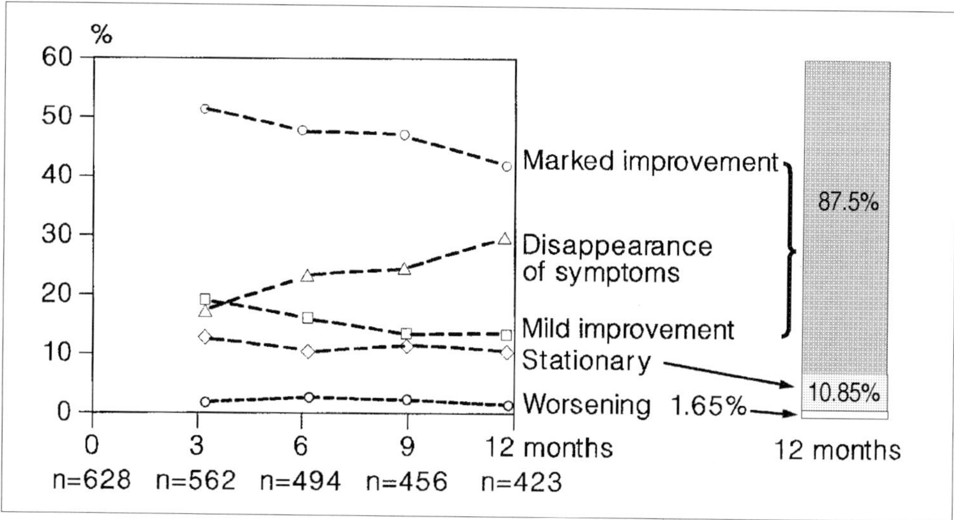

Figure 4. Long term open safety study : patient's overall evaluation of efficacy.

Quality of life is probably an important issue in functional disorders. However, no specific questionnaire has been validated for functional GI disorders. Since established questionnaires such as the Nottingham Health Profile and the General Well Being Index, used in the United Kingdom, were not sensitive enough to detect any significant difference between placebo and fedotozine, two additional questionnaires were administered in trials conducted in France. The former referred to as the Subjective Quality of Life Profile was able to detect a significant advantage in favour of fedotozine over placebo as well as metoclopramide in the phase III studies. Moreover, in a one-year open study, a number of items including food intake, pain and "digestion" were shown to improve from baseline to the end. The latter questionnaire designed by Chassany *et al.* is IBS-specific and was used in the phase III French study at an exploratory state and showed a significant improvement on fedotozine therapy as compared to placebo [5].

Safety

The withdrawals in all randomized trials with 30 mg t.i.d. or placebo were significantly more frequent on placebo than on fedotozine. Withdrawals for intercurrent events were not significantly different in both groups and withdrawals for loss to follow-up and lack of cooperation were also more frequent on placebo than on fedotozine. Pooling withdrawals for intercurrent event, treatment failure, loss to follow-up, lack of cooperation, *i.e.* withdrawals potentially treatment-related, a significant difference in favour of fedotozine arises, with a higher number of withdrawals on placebo.

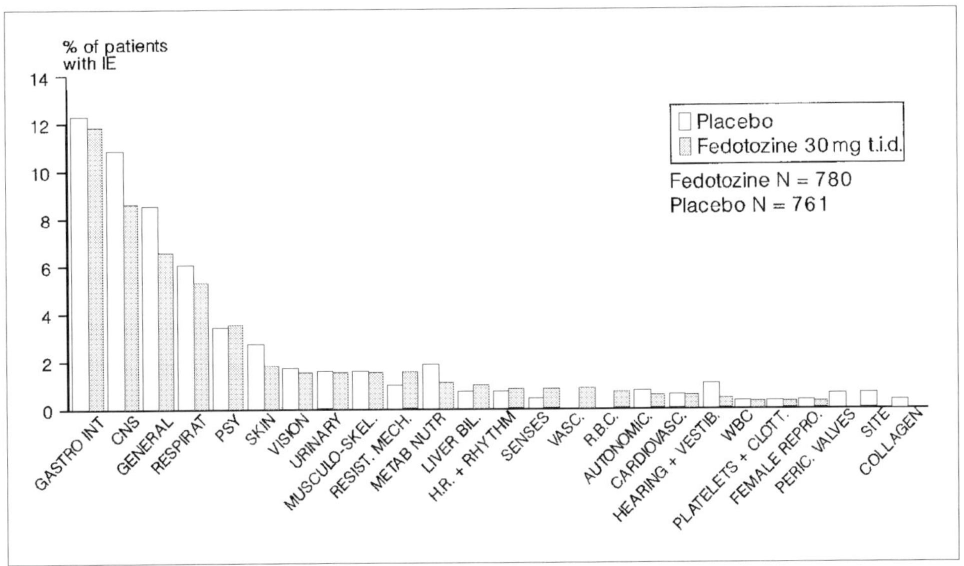

Figure 7. Intercurrent events in all studies including both a fedotozine 30 mg and a placebo group.

Finally the number of intercurrent events on fedotozine 30 mg t.i.d. and placebo, classified according to the various WHO body systems (Figure 5) was not different in any body system whatsoever, so that fedotozine seems to be extremely safe.

Conclusions

Taken together, these results indicate that fedotozine is a safe and effective drug in the treatment of functional disorders, especially FD and IBS. It compares well to existing drugs in FD and brings about a substantial benefit in terms of quality of life.

References

1. Fraitag B, Homerin M, Hecketsweiler P. Double-blind dose-response multicenter comparison of fedotozine and placebo in treatment of non ulcer dyspepsia. *Dig Dis Sci* 1994 ; 39 : 1072-7.
2. Galmiche JP, De Meynard C, Abitbol JL, Scherrer B, Fraitag B. Effects of fedotozine in chronic idiopathic dyspepsia : a double-blind placebo controlled multicentre study. *Gastroenterology* 1994 ; 106 : A502 (abstract).
3. Jian R, Abitbol JL, Scherrer B, Fraitag B. Fedotozine versus metoclopramide in functional dyspepsia : results of a 6 week multicenter therapeutic trial. *Gastroenterology* 1994 ; 106 : A518 (abstract).
4. Dapoigny M, Homerin M, Scherrer B, Fraitag B. Efficacy of fedotozine (F) in the irritable bowel syndrome (IBS). A double-blind placebo-controlled dose-range multicenter study. *Dig Dis Sci* 1995 (in press).

5. Chassany O, Genève J, Abitbol JL, Scherrer B, Dapoigny M, Fraitag B. Utilisation d'une nouvelle échelle de qualité de vie dans le syndrome de l'intestin irritable. Effet de la fedotozine. *Gastroenterol Clin Biol* 1995 ; 19 : A71 (abstract).

Sensitive gastrointestinal disorders. J.P. Galmiche, B. Fraitag.
John Libbey Eurotext, Paris © 1995, pp. 99-101

13

Effect of fedotozine in functional dyspepsia. A phase III double-blind placebo-controlled multicentre study

N.W. READ

Centre for Human Nutrition, Northern General Hospital, Sheffield, UK.

The aim of this multicentre study was to demonstrate the efficacy of fedotozine in the relief of symptoms in patients with functional dyspepsia (FD).

Methods

Three hundred and thirty patients were recruited by 25 hospital or GP centres within the United Kingdom and the Republic of Ireland. Of these, 271 (139 females and 132 males; age 42 years ± 14 years ; mean ± SD) fulfilled the entry criteria and were randomised to receive either fedotozine at a dose of 30 mg three times a day or an identical placebo given at the same frequency. One hundred and forty patients were randomised to receive fedotozine and 131 were randomised to receive placebo, and there were no significant difference in symptoms after randomisation.

The inclusion criteria for the studies were at least two of the following symptoms : inability to finish a normal meal, postprandial epigastric fullness/bloating, nausea or vomiting, feeling of slow digestion, epigastric pain. To be included, the patients had to have these symptoms for more than three months and at a frequency of at least three times a week. In addition, each patient had received a routine clinical work-up which included an upper gastrointestinal endoscopy and *Helicobacter* status, biliary ultrasonography and a routine blood test. Patients with any other severe illness, those under 18 or above 75 years of age, pregnant patients, patients taking any treatment potentially acting on the gastrointestinal tract, non-steroidal anti-inflammatory agents or neuroleptic agents or antidepressants were excluded from the study. Permitted treatments included beta blockers, nitrates, laxatives, adsorbants, antiflatulants, anxiolytics, fibre or bran, provided these were taken at a constant dose.

The study design was a double-blind, randomised trial of fedotozine 30 mg t.i.d. against an identical placebo. After a run-in period of one to two weeks, treatments were conducted for six weeks. Patients kept a diary of their symptoms throughout and were seen at the onset of the trial, after three weeks and after six weeks. The main assessment criterion was the diary of overall intensity of dyspeptic symptoms assessed on a guided analogue scale from none to slight, to moderate, to severe, and to very severe. Secondary criteria included a diary of individual dyspeptic symptoms kept in the same way and an investigator's assessment on a standard questionnaire. Any adverse events were recorded and biochemical/haematological indices were determined before and after treatment.

This was an intention-to-treat analysis and ANCOVA was carried out on the mean treatment effect over six weeks using the baseline as the covariate.

Results

Treatment with both placebo and fedotozine reduced the overall intensity of dyspeptic symptoms. The effect of fedotozine was significantly greater than the effect of placebo (p = 0.002). The response to fedotozine is shown more clearly in the time course in which a clear separation is seen between fedotozine and placebo after the first week of treatment. At the end of six weeks, there was a 70% reduction in overall intensity of symptoms. In addition to the overall effect, there were also significant improvements in epigastric pain on placebo compared with fedotozine. Sensation of fullness almost achieved significance as well (Table I).

The investigator's assessment failed to show any significant benefit of fedotozine and fedotozine did not appear to have any significant impact on quality of life assessment.

Adverse events

There were 23 adverse events leading to withdrawal, 13 on fedotozine, 10 on placebo. The only severely life threatening event was a case of pneumonia in the fedotozine group, though this was a patient who already had a low white count and the

Table I. Phase III study *versus* placebo (mean ± SD).

	Fedotozine n = 138		Placebo n = 131		p
Main criterion					
- run-in	1.58 ± 0.68		1.48 ± 0.68		
- treatment	1.14 ± 0.71	- 28%	1.24 ± 0.78	- 16%	0.002
Epigastric pain					
- run-in	1.25 ± 0.84		1.20 ± 0.83		
- treatment	0.87 ± 0.81	- 30%	1.00 ± 0.86	- 17%	0.004
Inability to finish a meal					
- run-in	0.84 ± 0.80		0.71 ± 0.80		
- treatment	0.66 ± 0.76	- 21%	0.59 ± 0.73	- 17%	0.592
Nausea					
- run-in	0.73 ± 0.76		0.62 ± 0.81		
- treatment	0.52 ± 0.71	- 29%	0.56 ± 0.74	- 10%	0.010
Slow digestion					
- run-in	1.17 ± 0.86		1.20 ± 0.80		
- treatment	0.86 ± 0.74	- 26%	0.96 ± 0.77	- 20%	0.157
Fullness					
-run-in	1.42 ± 0.75		1.38 ± 0.83		
-treatment	0.98 ± 0.75	- 26%	1.07 ± 0.84	- 22%	0.052
Patient's global score					
- run-in	1.08 ± 0.62		1.02 ± 0.62		
- treatment	0.78 ± 0.62	- 28%	0.84 ± 0.63	- 18%	0.021

Patient's global score = mean of the 5 symptoms.

p : Ancova (with run-in as the covariate).

% values : relative improvements $\frac{\text{(treatment-run-in)}}{\text{run-in}}$.

causality of fedotozine was doubtful. There were no significant abnormalities in biochemistry or haematology.

Conclusion

The efficacy of fedotozine is superior to that of placebo for the symptomatic relief of FD as assessed by the patients and the safety of fedotozine in this trial was excellent.

Sensitive gastrointestinal disorders. J.P. Galmiche, B. Fraitag.
John Libbey Eurotext, Paris © 1995, pp. 103-106

14

Efficacy of fedotozine in the irritable bowel syndrome. A double-blind placebo controlled dose-range multicentre study

M. DAPOIGNY, M. HOMERIN**, B. SCHERRER**, B. FRAITAG***

**Service de gastroentérologie, Hôtel Dieu, Clermont-Ferrand, France.*
***Institut de Recherche Jouveinal, Fresnes, France.*

Irritable bowel syndrome (IBS) is associated with altered visceral sensitivity and / or altered colonic or intestinal motility [1-4]. Up to now, no drug has been shown of benefit in the treatment of IBS. Fedotozine is a new κ 1-a-agonist [5-7] with several pharmacological effects in different animal models of pain or nociception with or without inflammation of the colonic mucosa (*see previous chapters*). Our aim was therefore to access the efficacy and safety of fedotozine as compared to placebo in a multicentre controlled study.

Methods

Patients were recruited in different centres in France, Belgium and Tunisia. Among 313 eligible patients, 238 were randomized either to fedotozine or placebo. The selection criterion was abdominal pain which had to be accompanied by one or more

Manning's criteria, the latter including in particular diarrhoea and/or constipation, and bloating [8]. The symptoms had to be present for more than one year. In addition, work-up for organic gastrointestinal disease had to be negative. History, clinical examination, upper gastrointestinal endoscopy and ultrasonography had to be found normal.

According to the study design (Figure 1), the patients had to take one tablet of placebo t.i.d. for two weeks, and, at the end of a 2-week period, if they were still meeting the selection criteria, they could be randomized to one of the four groups, *i.e.* placebo 3.5 mg fedotozine t.i.d., 15 mg fedotozine t.i.d., and 30 mg t.i.d., for six weeks with an interim assessment. The main criterion was the maximal intensity of abdominal pain as recorded by the patient on a diary, four times a day, as very severe, severe, moderate, mild or absent.

The secondary assessment criteria included the mean daily abdominal pain, the mean intensity of bloating, and bowel habits and defecation disorders, all these being derived from the same diary. Finally, the patients had to assess the overall efficacy of the treatment. The investigators had to rate the overall intensity of IBS and the overall efficacy of the treatment. We also evaluated the safety of the treatment by clinical examination, biology and ECG. Intention-to-treat statistical analysis was peformed using polynomial contrasts between time and treatments while the safety was evaluated by ANOVA.

A significant decrease in intensity of maximal daily pain was observed with fedotozine as compared to placebo, only at 30 mg t.i.d., particularly during the last three weeks of treatment. As shown in Figure 2, fedotozine was also superior to placebo in

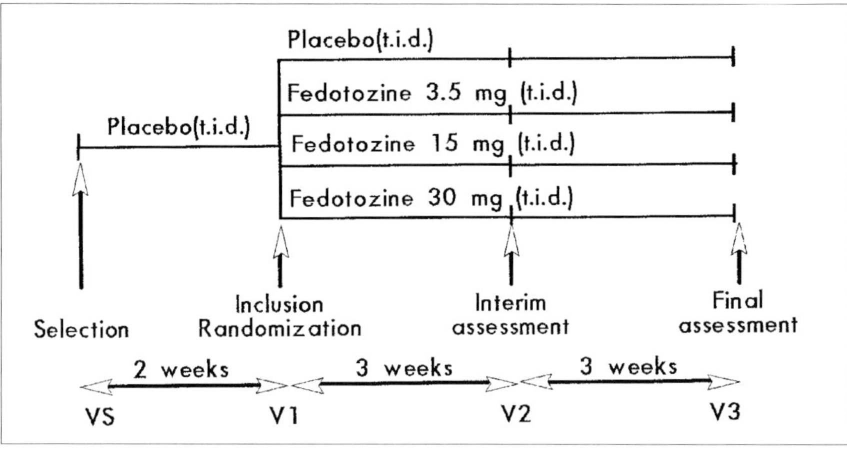

Figure 1. Study design. The selected patients received, for a two week run-in period, a placebo t.i.d. and then were randomized to one of the four treatment groups. The treatment phase was divided into two therapeutic periods of three weeks separated by an interim evaluation.

terms of days without pain, thus resulting in a 129% improvement as compared to 72% on placebo (p =0.021).

Among second criteria, the mean daily pain (expressed as the variation from baseline) was also statistically improved by fedotozine 30 mg t.i.d. *versus* placebo (p < 0.007). Accordingly bloating was relieved to a higher extent by fedotozine (p < 0.02 *versus* placebo).

Regarding the patient's assessment of the overall efficacy of the treatment, the global test did not show any significant difference between the four groups. However, there was a high proportion of patients with markedly improved sensation during treatment with 3.5 mg and 30 mg fedotozine, respectively 50% and 46% compared to 29% on placebo. Bowel habits and defecation disorders were not assessable in this study, probably because the patients poorly understood this section of their diaries. When assessed by the investigators, fedotozine significantly improved the overall severity of IBS at 30 mg t.i.d. (p<0.003). Fedotozine, at the same dosage, improved the pain component of the symptom profile (p<0.009), and the overall treatment efficacy was also statistically significant (p<0.02).

Safety was good, no serious side effect being recorded during the study. There were no intergroup differences in the number of side effects appearance and withdrawals for side effects in the four groups. Final biological essessment and ECG were normal on completion of the study.

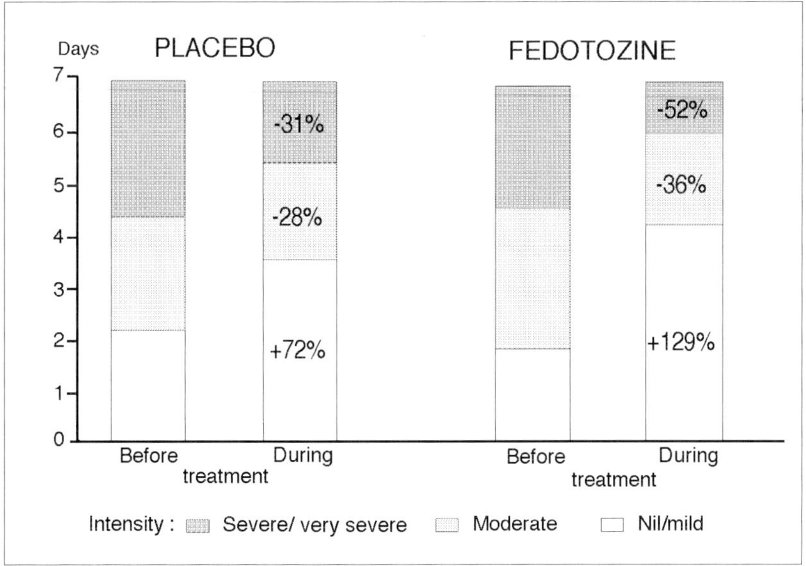

Figure 2. Main criterion. Abdominal pain before and during treatment. Number of days (per week) at each intensity level (ITT).

In conclusion, in this phase II study, fedotozine was safe at all dosages. Fedotozine 30 mg t.i.d. was effective on abdominal pain in IBS as assessed by the patients and the investigators. The results are further supported by another multicentre study performed according to the same trial design and aiming at the comparison of fedotozine 30 mg t.i.d. with placebo. Indeed there was a significant improvement of pain in the fedotozine group over placebo. Should these first results be confirmed in further studies, fedotozine seems a promising drug for the treatment of IBS.

References

1. Lind CD. Motility disorders in the irritable bowel syndrome. *Gastroenterol Clin North Am* 1991 ; 20 : 279-95.
2. Ritchie J. Pain from distension of the pelvic colon by inflating a balloon in the irritable colon syndrome. *Gut* 1973 ; 14 : 125-32.
3. Read NW. Irritable bowel syndrome (IBS), definition and pathophysiology. *Scand J Gastroenterol* 1987 ; 130 (suppl.) : 7-13.
4. Wingate DL. The irritable bowel syndrome. *Gastroenterol Clin North Am* 1991 ; 20 : 351-62.

5. Rivière PJM, Pascaud X, Chevalier E, Le Gallou B, Junien JL. Fedotozine reverses ileus induced by surgery or peritonitis : action at peripheral κ–opioid receptors. *Gastroenterology* 1993 ; 104 : 724-31.
6. Gué M, Junien JL, Pascaud X, Buéno L. Antagonism of stress-induced motor alterations and plasma cortisol release by fedotozine (JO 1196) in dogs. *J Gastrointest Motil* 1990 ; 2 : 258-64.
7. Coffin J, Jian R, Lémann M, Fraitag B, Van Egroo LD, Franchisseur C, Rambaud JC. Fedotozine increases threshold of discomfort to gastric distension in healthy subjects. *Gastroenterology* 1992 ; 102 : A437 (abstract).
8. Manning AP, Thompson WG, Heaton KW, Lorris AF. Towards positive diagnosis of the irritable bowel. *Br Med J* 1978 ; 2 : 653-4.

Sensitive gastrointestinal disorders. J.P. Galmiche, B. Fraitag.
John Libbey Eurotext, Paris © 1995, pp. 107-108

Conclusion

J.P. GALMICHE

Service d'Hépato-Gastroentérologie, Hôpital Guillaume et René Laënnec, 44035 Nantes Cedex 01, France.

Gastrointestinal functional disorders are thought to be responsible for many symptoms encountered by general practitioners and gastroenterologists as well. After two decades of active research in the field of GI motility, it has become more and more obvious that a significant proportion of those patients seeking medical help have an altered visceral perception rather than a motility disturbance.

Most of the evidence supporting this concept of abnormal pain perception was critically reviewed during the first session of this symposium. Of interest is the fact that new tools (*e.g.* barostat) are now available for human studies and that rigorous protocols with more objective assessment criteria have been recently defined.

In that context, the discovery of kappa opioid receptors constituted an important landmark and pointed towards a new direction for control of nociception and visceral pain. Moreover, it has now been established that kappa receptors exist in different subtypes and that the kappa 1 receptor includes two subtypes K_{1A} and K_{1B}. Fedotozine, a new compound developed by the Institut de Recherche Jouveinal, has been shown to act primarily at the K_{1A} receptor. This finding explains why fedotozine, unlike other kappa ligands, does not display psychotomimetic adverse effects or does not produce diuresis. This unique pharmocological profile seems extremely promising since functional dyspepsia or irritable bowel syndrome, while being non life-threatening conditions, are responsible for disabling symptoms. Therefore a drug active in functional disorders should relieve pain but should not induce central nervous system symptom effects, urinary retention or incontinence and moreover should not result in psychological or physical dependence. Contrary to other opioid agonists, many evidences are presented in this book that fedotozine acts at the peripheral level by reducing or blocking the function of afferent fibers.

Interestingly, several elegant models have been described and can now be employed as *in vivo* tests of potency and efficiency including, for example, models of irritation and inflammation in animals and sleep deprivation in humans. Taken together, the data presented during the Versailles symposium provide an excellent rationale for the development of fedotozine, and more generally speaking of K_{1A} ligands in the treatment of functional disorders and visceral pain. Accordingly, during the last session of this meeting, the results of well-designed clinical trials conducted in several European countries were first reported in details. It is fair to congratulate Jouveinal researchers for being able to enrol a large number of patients with functional dyspepsia or irritable bowel syndrome in these trials and to develop specific tools for the assessment of parameters of pivotal importance as quality of life. As expected from pre-clinical experiments, most of these therapeutic trials strongly support a benefit of fedotozine in both functional dyspepsia and irritable bowel syndrome. Moreover, the available data clearly establish the safety profile of the drug, even in the long term.

Finally, the therapeutic advance made with fedotozine should be put in perspective with the other existing drugs in the field of GI functional disorders. This drug may represent the leader compound of a new and very promising pharmacological class. That's where we are ! But now where should we go ? Regarding basic concepts, it seems quite clear that additional research is urgently requested to further elucidate the molecular and cellular mechanisms of action of kappa ligands and to define the specific target receptor required for pharmacological activity. On the other hand, clinical trials should be encouraged with fedotozine or with the following compounds that pharmaceutical companies and especially Jouveinal may have in the pipeline. Regarding these trials to be performed in dyspepsia or irritable bowel syndrome, it seems also an appropriate time to develop guidelines concerning study design and to try to define the specific subgroups than may or may not respond to the different types of drugs thought to act on either motility or visceral pain perception (or both). Assessment criteria relevant to clinical use, including quality of life, are probably an important part of these recommendations, which are of course beyond the scope of this symposium.

Achevé d'imprimer par   Corlet, Imprimeur, S.A.
14110 Condé-sur-Noireau (France)
N° d'Imprimeur : 12386 - Dépôt légal : septembre 1995

Imprimé en C.E.E.